Beyond Hot And Crazy

The Radical Guide to Living Well With Menopause

By

Pam Lob

Foreword by Rachel Jayne Groover,
Bestselling Author of Powerful and Feminine

Deep
Pacific
Press

Beyond Hot and Crazy
The Radical Guide to Living Well With Menopause

Copyright © 2017 Pamela Lob.

First edition: Balboa Press February 2015

Second Edition: Deep Pacific Press November 2017

Editor: Karen Collyer https://www.karencollyer.com/
Images: Courtesy of Inspirational Nature Pictures

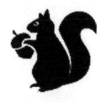

This book is dedicated to the
Regal Squirrel Chicks
Amara
Miyuki
Pat
Lisa
Thank you for your love, support and belief in me.

xxx

INVITATION FROM THE AUTHOR

Throughout this book there are interactive opportunities in the form of video's. Mp3's and documents to support you in reading this book and in transforming your health and life.

FREE Additional Resources

- Instant Tips to Move Beyond Hot and Crazy PDF
- Healthy Eating Hypnotherapy MP3
- Emotional Release and Destress Hypnotherapy MP3
- Seaside Walk Meditation MP3

Download at
http://beyondhotcrazy.gr8.com/

Hooray. This book is interactive with videos, meditations and other resources to deepen your experience. Scan the QR codes with a code reader or your phone camera to be taken directly to the resource or just type the url into your browser. Enjoy.

FOREWORD
BY RACHEL JAYNE GROOVER

Presence is the key to mastering all aspects of your life. It starts with actively reconnecting with your body, and then understanding how you feel. Once you do that, you can fully access, trust, and express your inner 'knowing,' and actively choose to take steps that are in alignment with this wisdom.

Working with women from around the world, I am acutely aware of how deeply we are impacted by our disconnection from our bodies and our feminine essence. We often numb ourselves to feeling our body and emotions, which leaves us unsure of how to access our own inner wisdom.

This means we tend to rely on others to guide our decisions and make our lifestyle choices. This seems to be more pronounced during menopause, as often many aspects of a woman's life change in profound ways during those years, and we turn to others for advice and wisdom.

In my work with the *Art of Feminine Presence*™ trainings, I am continually surrounded by women of all ages, which offers me a unique perspective on the life stages that we all go through sooner or later. One stage that is quite challenging for many women is menopause. It seems to me that there are a lot of misconceptions and beliefs that have not been questioned and explored and that promote expectations of this being a difficult time in life.

I don't believe it has to be this way. I look forward to this time in my life as much as to any other stage that is still ahead for me.

I appreciate the information that Pam provides in this book to help me make informed decisions on how best to maintain my health and energy as I move into menopause in the next few years. It is a natural process — not a medical one — and with the right lifestyle choices, can be traversed with minimal or no discomfort.

I first met Pam Lob at an event four years ago and she was one of those women who reported that she felt disconnected, unsure and overwhelmed by life. I've witnessed her rapid transformation in her physical, mental, and spiritual health as she began to reconnect with her feminine essence and learned to listen and trust herself in a new and deeper way. She has since established herself as a leader and has a joyous, caring and engaging presence that is lovely to be around.

This book is the result of her journey, her struggles and her successes. She offers insights into some of the most commonly held myths and negative beliefs surrounding menopause while offering natural, empowered and proactive solutions that can easily and effectively be integrated into your everyday life.

Blessings on your journey through this transformational phase of your life.

Rachael Jayne Groover

Creator of *Art of Feminine Presence*™

Author of *Powerful and Feminin*

Table of Contents

Introduction – Menopause
A time to dread, or A time to rejoice?

"A study says owning a dog makes you 10 years younger. My first thought was to rescue two more, but I don't want to go through menopause again".
Joan Rivers

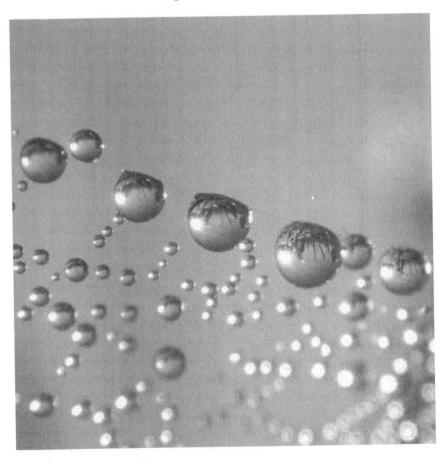

Menopause

A Time to Dread, Or A Time to Rejoice?

There are thousands, if not millions of women struggling daily with symptoms blamed on menopause. They feel embarrassed and mortified by hot flushes that occur at inopportune moments. They find it hard to sleep, or even worse wake steaming and soaked in sweat.

Brain fog makes it difficult to concentrate at work and they find themselves snapping at colleagues and loved ones for no real reason. If they consult a doctor, their symptoms are often blamed on menopause and they are offered Hormone Replacement Therapy (HRT) and anti-depressants. Few doctors bother to look at the real causes of their patient's symptoms.

Menopause is something all women go through, but it's rarely discussed. It feels like a taboo subject. Women have no one to turn to and share experiences with, as friends and colleagues are also suffering in silence.

Menopause is a time of their lives that many women dread, or at least see as a time to endure. I am on a mission to change that. I want all women to see their mid-life as a time to rejoice and to connect with themselves, not a time of struggle and being at the beck and call of their families and careers.

There is no reason why women cannot feel healthy, radiant and alive, looking forward to the second half of their lives.

I wish I could tell you that all you need to do is wave a magic wand and hey presto, everything is all right with you and the world. But there is no magical quick fix.

So...

This book is about **living**, learning to live your life to the full, making the most of opportunities and finding joy in all moments, no matter what.

This book is for you if you are a woman who:

- Has menopausal symptoms and want to go through this time of your life naturally and empowered.

- Is proactive and wants to prepare and prevent menopause symptoms occurring.

- Want practices and strategies that can become part of your daily routine.

- Want to transform your life for the better, not just during menopause, but also beyond.

- Are ready to implement changes in your life so you can feel healthier and more joyful and as a result, have better relationships with yourself and others.

Menopause is a natural phenomenon not a medical one, though the medical profession wants you to believe otherwise! Often doctors will look at your symptoms and blame them on the catchword of menopause without going to the root cause of your symptoms.

You are unique and therefore your menopause is specific to you. Many symptoms blamed on menopause are due to something else. A woman with a healthy and balanced life will experience none, or only slight menopausal symptoms.

I want to share with you what I've discovered on my journey, so you can have an easy, natural transition into the second half of your life.

My belief, gained from extensive research and my experience, is that the primary causes of menopausal symptoms are:

- Stress

- Diet

- Chemicals and toxins in your environment

- Limiting beliefs

- Disconnection from your body, emotions, energy and feminine essence.

My aim is to:

- Present a holistic viewpoint for each of these topics, meaning that you are paying attention to your body, mind, emotions, energy and spirit, plus your relationships, work and play.

- Give you detailed information, so you can make informed decisions from a place of knowledge and clarity.

- Offer easy to implement tips and practices that help you deal with those pesky menopausal symptoms.

- Support you in having a healthy, joyous life, that will benefit both you and your loved ones, for now and the rest of your days.

If you read this book and continue just as you have been doing, then nothing will change. It's up to you to make the choice and begin taking small action steps towards a new life today

My Story

Watch: My Story
http://www.pamlob.com/my-story/

For most of my life I have battled with hormonal and gynecological issues. I always felt unheard, misunderstood and let down by the medical profession around my own problems. From the age of fifteen, I experienced chronic pelvic pain, not always associated with my periods, which were always something to be endured. Whenever I visited my doctor (GP), I was told things like:

"You have a grumbling appendix."

"It's just irritable bowel syndrome."

"You're a woman, what do you expect?"

"You're on the pill, so it can't be that bad!"

"Just take paracetamol and get on with what you need to do."

As a qualified nurse, in my early thirties I still thought that the medical profession had all the answers, if you found the right doctor. But as I struggled with my pain and trying to discover what was behind it, I came to realise that they didn't.

To cope with what was now severe pain for most of the month, whilst also having the capacity to care for two young children, I explored complementary therapies.

A friend recommended reflexology. Oh no I couldn't have someone tickling my feet! But when you are desperate you are prepared to try anything. To begin with, I was sceptical and believed all reflexology did was help me relax. How could points on my feet tell me anything about my health? However, after visiting my reflexologist a few times, she said, "I believe all your symptoms are caused by endometriosis and I recommend that you to go back to see your doctor."

I wasn't even sure what endometriosis was. It has only been in the last few years that endometriosis has begun to be recognized as a possible cause of women's pelvic pain, without years of suggesting it is something else.

My GP was doubtful when I said I thought my symptoms were due to endometriosis. I suspect he didn't know much about it either. With reluctance he agreed to refer me to a gynecologist.

Finally, at the age of thirty-six, a diagnosis of endometriosis was confirmed after a laparoscopy. It was a huge relief to get a diagnosis and find out I wasn't going mental!

My reflexologist turned out to be correct and I will be forever grateful. She could help me with my symptoms more than anyone else. I was no longer a sceptic but became a convert who now recommends reflexology to all her clients. I was able to see that reflexology not only helped me relax, but also helped balance my hormones and boost my immune system. I'm sure it was my weekly sessions that kept me functioning as a mother and wife.

Over the next few years the pain became worse and worse. Some days I'd drive to pick up the kids from school, gripping the steering wheel as hard as I could, as I experienced waves of intense pain. Painkillers did little to help, other than make me feel sick, dizzy and unable to function. It felt like being drunk and hung over at the same time. Not something I would recommend! So I gave up taking them.

My gynecologist tried various treatments including Zoladex injections and the Marina coil, which both led to hot flushes and other menopausal symptoms. The hardest to deal with, other than the pain, was the constant overwhelming fatigue. What I wanted was the energy to do whatever I wanted. It wasn't until years later, when I was fifty-five and the first edition of this book published, that I had my wish fully materialise.

During this time I tried various treatments suggested by my gynecologist. I also researched deeper into alternative and complimentary therapies and experimented with anything I thought might bring relief. Within this book I will share those that worked for me and have also brought relief to my clients.

By the time I was forty, my gynecologist had run out of options to keep the pain under some control and recommended a total hysterectomy. This meant that at age forty I was tossed into a surgically induced menopause. I was strongly advised to start Hormone Replacement Therapy (HRT) and told that without it my menopausal symptoms would be unbearable. Doctors also warned me that without HRT I was at extremely high risk for osteoporosis and heart disease. I reluctantly agreed to HRT, but at the lowest dose possible. I used HRT patches at a dose given to women with fully functioning ovaries.

Post hysterectomy I felt amazing. Words can't do justice to how great it feels to be pain free. Yes, I was getting regular hot flushes and still struggled with fatigue, but nothing like I had felt pre-surgery.

The ongoing battle with my hormones and the constant fatigue led me on a journey of discovery about endometriosis and menopause. I learnt how to balance my hormones naturally through healthy eating, complementary therapies, self-care and connecting to who I am as a woman.

The most important piece of learning for me is to listen to what my body and my intuition is telling me it needs at any moment, rather than listening to the little nagging voice in my head.

As I write, it has been sixteen years since my hysterectomy. I've not taken HRT for twelve years. Along the way I gained the confidence to complete a degree in psychology, train as a Counsellor, Hypnotherapist, Heart Intelligence Coach, Personalised Health Coach and Art of Feminine Presence teacher.

I now feel fitter, healthier, more energised and younger than I did in my twenties.

I want the same for you and I'm looking forward to guiding you on your own journey through an exciting and empowering time of your life.

Setting the Stage
The Key to Your Extraordinary Life

When you do things from your soul, you feel a river moving in you, a joy.
Rumi

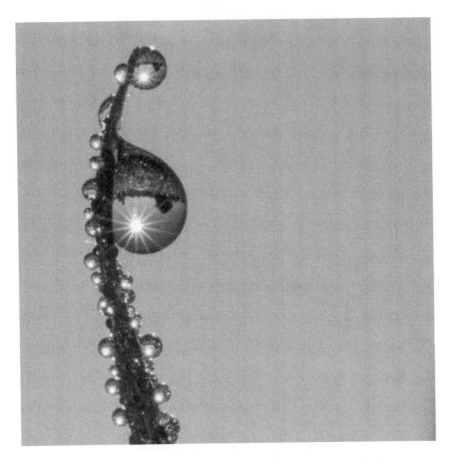

The Key to Your Extraordinary Life

Watch The Key to an Extraordinary Life
http://www.pamlob.com/key-extraordinary-life

As you read this book, I invite you to be open minded about what is possible. I want you to take a step back out of yourself to allow you to view things from a different perspective.

Life can be extraordinary when you connect with **who you are**, rather than being ruled by your normal limiting mindset, its stories and judgments, or by listening to what others say you should do.

I believe in quality of life and my greatest desire is for you to say, as you lie on your deathbed, "I had my ups and downs, but overall it was a great ride." In the words of Brendon Burchard:

"I lived, I loved, I mattered."

One day, our life on this earth will come to an end. Death is the only thing we can be certain of, yet none of us know how or when. When I was nursing, I cared for people who were told they only had a limited time to live. Some were given six months to live, yet lived for many years longer. Some of those people are still here today, fit and well. I also know of people who have died for no particular reason, other than they had given up the will to live.

You have the choice whether your life is just plain ordinary, or whether it is extraordinary. We all have the opportunity and capabilities within us to lead an extraordinary life. Yet so many choose to play it safe, follow the crowd and become disconnected from their body, emotions and essence. They put up with what life throws at them, including menopausal symptoms.

The dictionary definition of ordinary is, "with no special or distinctive features; normal."

Unfortunately, many women think of menopausal symptoms as normal!

Many women find themselves stuck in a rut, leading ordinary lives that often seem as though they are stuck in 'Groundhog Day,' doing the same thing day in day out. They rush around each morning getting the kids ready for school, themselves ready for work, dropping the kids off, working all day, then rushing home. Time then to sort out homework, housework and supper, reaching out for a glass or two of wine in the belief it helps them survive...

Just writing this feels exhausting and I remember vividly my life being like this!

Does this sound like you as well?

Even if you don't have children, or they have flown the nest, the constant struggle of balancing work and home life is a battle that many women are losing. The constant rush from one thing to another, constantly being at someone else's beck and call, leads to stress, overwhelm and feelings of disconnection from who you are.

There is nothing wrong with ordinary, but you deserve and are capable of so much more. You are extraordinary!

A great analogy to represent **YOU** is a water droplet. When you look at a drop of water, you can see its beauty and purity and notice it is whole. Just like **YOU**. You might not believe it because all you notice are challenges like, "I can barely walk, I constantly forget things, my husband has just left me."

I'm sure you can come up with a fairly big list of what you believe is wrong with you!

I am here to tell you **No,** there is nothing wrong with **YOU**.

Maybe part of your physical body isn't functioning optimally, or you're going through a difficult experience right now, but this doesn't define who you are.

One way to understand this concept is to imagine your problems as mud stirred into a glass of water. The water looks dirty and unfit to drink, but if you leave it to settle for a while, the particles of mud sink to the bottom of the glass, leaving clean, drinkable water on top.

11

Even with immense physical disabilities, it is possible to turn your life around and find joy, excitement, optimism and to feel connected to a sense of wholeness. Your life may not be what you dreamed of, or envisioned, but it can be just as fulfilling, if not more so.

Spencer West, a man from Toronto, Canada, had both legs amputated as a child but that hasn't stopped him from climbing Kilimanjaro. Nick Vujicic was born without arms and legs but this hasn't stopped him from becoming an amazing inspirational speaker, getting married and having a child. Tanni Grey-Thompson DBE was born with Spina Bifida and has spent her life in a wheel chair. This has not stopped her from winning sixteen Paralympic medals and the London Marathon six times. She is now a patron for various charities and sits in the House of Lords.

No matter what you see as wrong with you, there is always a way. Sometimes it requires more imagination and ingenuity to get there.

Another beautiful attribute of a water droplet is when you look at it in sunlight you can see a myriad of colours, just like a rainbow. I like to envision these colours as your emotions. If you take one colour away, there is no rainbow. Likewise, if you take away one of your emotions, you will not be complete.

Culture, society and upbringing have led many of us to believe certain emotions are wrong and shouldn't be expressed, or some emotions are negative and should be avoided at all cost!

When you repress an emotion, it becomes stuck in your body as a cellular memory, until one day you've accumulated so much pressure and tension it erupts like a pressure cooker letting off a build-up of steam. This manifests as cancer, heart disease, chronic illnesses, or you have an accident that makes you take time out.

Cellular memory can be a cause of menopausal symptoms. Along with subconscious limiting beliefs, it can affect how you will transition through the menopause.

The secret is learning to accept what you are feeling right now and how to release your emotions safely. This does not mean you must like what you are feeling, instead just allow yourself to 'be'. I will teach you how to do this throughout this book.

I believe we have two options on how we choose to live our lives, doing nothing, or taking action. Imagining yourself as a water droplet. Would you rather spend your time in a pond of murky everyday experiences, like being stuck in an endless 'Groundhog Day', or would you leap into the 'River of Life' where you can stretch and discover your possibilities?

This book is an invitation for you to explore and discover new ideas and try on new practices.

Are you ready to join me in the 'River of Life'?

From a Pond to the River of Life

As I look back at my life, it feels as though I spent a large part of it living in a pond of mediocrity. As ponds go, it was in a nice neighbourhood, surrounded by nature, but the banks were made up of my severely limiting beliefs. My disconnection from my body, emotions, energy and intuition kept me swimming in circles and playing small.

Over time, due to my health issues, I began to feel the limitations of the pond and started to explore what else was possible. This is when I discovered the river. I began to slowly dip my toes in and sometimes even spent a whole week there, only to rush back to the safety of the pond.

At the end of 2003 my husband was diagnosed with leukaemia and had to undergo chemotherapy, which involved spending weeks at a time in hospital.

Suddenly I was catapulted straight into the river, into the rapids! We never knew what each day would bring and sometimes it was living a minute at a time. One minute we were meandering gently through the water meadows, then the next minute we were catapulted back into the rapids, or free-falling down a waterfall.

Living in the river felt very scary at times, but I discovered, to my amazement, it was also very joyful, satisfying and rewarding.

13

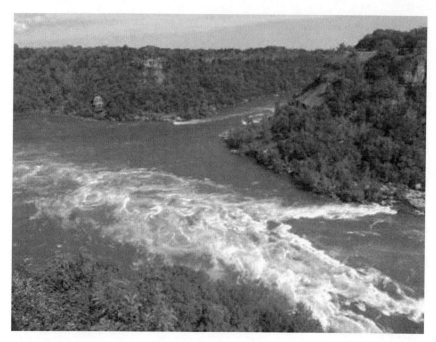

My husband and I spent large amounts of time together in his small hospital room. It could have been boring, but it wasn't. It gave us the opportunity to learn to connect with each other more deeply and to appreciate the simple things in life.

All around us others were flailing in the water, waiting and hoping that somebody would throw them a lifejacket, rather than living in the moment and finding enjoyment in the ride. Even in the dark moments there is joy if you're prepared to open your eyes and see.

When my husband died a year later, I had learnt to live in the river and this gave me strength as I dealt with my grief and came to terms with being a single parent.

It is much better to learn to live in the 'River of Life' when you can take the time and choose to be there, rather than be catapulted in by a major problem or event.

The final chapter of this book gives you several strategies that will help you live in the 'River of Life' and be extraordinary. I've tried to put everything in an order that I believe will give you the most benefit. You can dip in and out of the final chapter from the start.

As stress is a major factor in causing menopausal symptoms and overwhelm is a big part of many lives, I suggest working on just one strategy at a time. Once you are comfortable with the ideas and are implementing them into your daily life, add the next one.

Remember it can take up to ninety days for something to become a habit, so please be patient.

So… are you ready?

Take my hand and let me lead you into the 'River of Life.'

Join the River of Life

Listen and download
River of Life Meditation
http://www.pamlob.com/river-of-life/

Settle down in a comfortable, quiet place and take your focus to your breath.

Take three easy breaths, letting the air sink right down into your belly and then exhale slowly through your mouth. Let your muscles relax, especially your jaw.

Now imagine yourself as a little water droplet, floating around a pond seeing the same scenery every day, coming across the same stories, beliefs and experiences that are preventing you from having the life of your dreams.

Now imagine one day, warmed by the sun, you can leave the safety of your pond and float up effortlessly to join a big white fluffy cloud in a brilliant blue sky. Enjoy the freedom of floating without a care or worry. Look down on the beautiful earth below and all the different experiences available to you.

Eventually you fall genteelly as rain into a river, the wonderful 'River of Life.'

The river is your heart, your energy and your lifeblood. The scenery that you are flowing through represents your emotions and the movement of the water helps you to feel these emotions.

You are able to feel, really feel, for the first time since being a young child. You feel all the other water droplets around you, the warmth of the sun or the cold of the night, the power of the water's flow, sometimes gentle and soothing, other times bumpy, wild and frightening.

You may be meandering through the water meadows feeling calm, peaceful, and happy. You may find yourself in a mountainous area, with rapids that make you feel pain, fear and anger as water droplets constantly barge into you. But then one of these droplets takes your hand and tells you not to be afraid, as you'll continue this journey together, supporting each other, and your emotion changes to love.

You come to a waterfall and depending on how you are feeling as you go over the edge, your reaction may be, "Aghhhhh, help!!!!!" or, "Weeeeee, wow this is great!!!!!" As you get to the bottom of the waterfall, the power of the water behind you catapults you into the air. It feels so good to fly and the sun shines through you, showing you as a rainbow - whole, perfect and with a complete range of emotions.

Sometimes you may find yourself stuck behind a rock, or in an area of still water. You feel like you did back in the pond, with thoughts preventing you from feeling. The little voice in

16

your head telling you not to continue down the river, as there may be more rapids, waterfalls or even crocodiles.

But you now know how joyful it is to experience life to the full and you know that all it takes to get back into the stream of life is to move. Maybe slowly, sensuously or maybe more energetically, through the use of sound, "Mmmmmmmmmmm" or "Ohhhhh" or by asking for help from someone passing.

And the journey continues, sometimes fun and exhilarating, sometimes rough and painful and sometimes smooth, calm and relaxing. You may stay in this river or you may join a cloud and fall gently as snow, or as hard as hail into another river, another place, so that you expand your life experiences, your emotions, your feelings more and more.

Take three deep breaths and sit quietly for a few minutes contemplating how different your life will be in the beautiful 'River of Life.'

If there is something in this book that you don't understand, or want support with, please do not hesitate to contact me:

http://www.pamlob.com/contact

CHAPTER 1

How to Understand Your Raging Hormones!

The wound is the place where the Light enters you.
Rumi

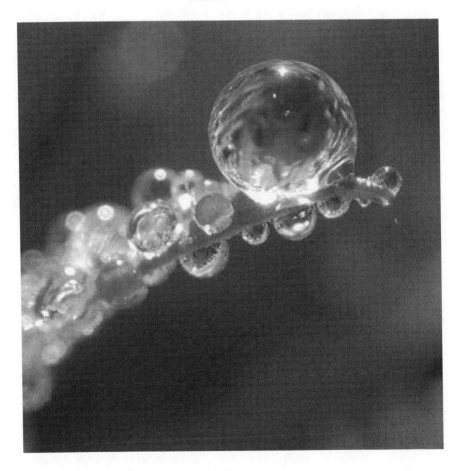

HOW TO UNDERSTAND YOUR RAGING HORMONES!

Watch How to Understand your Raging Hormones
http://www.pamlob.com/understand raging
hormones

> *"I feel like someone has put me in an oven."*

> *"I've turned into a total bitch! I've reached the point where I don't even like the person I have become."*

> *"I feel weak, exhausted, shut off and alone".*

These are three of many comments I hear time and again from women going through the menopause. Do you resonate with these?

Midlife transition in the past and for a few cultures today is a time for women to celebrate, to leave the responsibility of childbearing years behind and enter a phase of creativity and wisdom. However, today due to the use of contraception many women delay childbearing until later in life. They dread the onset of menopause and the loss of their dream to have a child, or another child. In a twist of fate, menopause is starting at a younger and younger age. Another repercussion of having children at a later age is they can end up struggling with menopause at the same time as their children are experiencing the ups and downs of puberty. The result hormonal fireworks!

Women today have become disconnected from their femininity as they take on a male persona from an early age to survive in school and the workplace, which are organised from a predominantly male orientation. And thanks to the media the image of being feminine is all about looks, being thin and tall like a model, wearing beautiful clothes, with a face plastered in makeup.

It has become normal for women to be working full time, whilst also caring for a home and family, plus as they reach menopause ageing parents. As a result, many women today see menopause as a time to dread, a time of loss and struggle with health, difficult emotions and low energy. They are left wondering what the hell is going on. It feels like they are losing control of their bodies and lives!

We are led to believe most, if not all women, struggle with the menopause, experience hot flushes, weight gain and loss of sex drive.

This is a myth perpetuated by the medical profession, pharmaceutical industry and the media. Even here in the western world, there are many women who have none, or only minor difficulties. Several women I've spoken to as I've been writing this book have reacted with surprise to discover that menopause causes such difficulty for other women. Many others have told me tales of woe and embarrassment, believing that menopause truly sucks. Very few share openly with other women and family members how they feel.

Research suggests that around 70% of women in the western world suffer some symptoms deemed to be due to menopause.

This is huge and a large proportion of them are having a really torrid time, yet like many other women's health issues menopause is rarely openly discussed!

Menopause typically happens in the late forties too early fifties, with early menopause occurring before the age of forty-five. The number of women experiencing early menopause is on the increase, with some reporting symptoms in their mid-thirties. The women who often struggle the most are those who have had a surgical menopause due to hysterectomy. This involves the removal of the uterus and in a total hysterectomy, the ovaries too. These women are also frequently young to experience menopause and have had none, or barely any perimenopause, so their body has had no time to adjust.

However, it's not a foregone conclusion that women will have a horrendous time post hysterectomy. I felt much healthier after my hysterectomy, despite being on the lowest dose of HRT possible. Hot flushes were a nuisance, but I'd been having them for some time anyway.

Others have said the same thing. Probably because the reason they had needed a hysterectomy in the first place had caused them to feel so rotten, menopausal symptoms were quite a breeze in comparison. This was certainly true for me.

In the past the majority of women sailed through menopause with little discomfort, today about eighty percent of women in the west report experiencing at least some menopausal symptoms. However some cultures have no problems with menopause, instead seeing it as a time for sexual freedom without the fear of getting pregnant. It is a time for connection and knowing of self, rather than having to concentrate on other's needs, as children become independent. In some languages there are not even words to describe this time of life.

Some argue that true feminine power does not fully bloom until we reach the power stage of life, which is midlife onwards. Research shows that there is a major spike in a woman's creativity aged fifty, that can last for twenty-five to thirty years. In the past and in some tribes today, the matriarchal elder woman is celebrated and revered by all, including the warriors, for her knowledge and intuition.

In western culture today there is an obsession with youth. The media and the medical profession, encouraged by large pharmaceutical companies, are constantly pushing pills, potions and cosmetics that will keep us looking forever young, or at least striving for the unavailable elixir of youth.

Along with the toxicity of our environment and disconnection from self and nature, women are permanently stressed and stopped from reaching their true power and potential.

What is Menopause?

Menopause, like puberty, is a natural phenomenon that all women will go through at some stage. It isn't a sudden stopping of menstruation, but a gradual process of change to hormone levels involved in fertility. You are deemed to be menopausal one year after the cessation of any menstrual bleed.

It could be argued menopause is 'just a day'! Before this day you are perimenopausal and after post-menopausal.

The time leading up to menopause is known as the perimenopause. It's the time that your hormones are going through the transitional phase leading up to menopause. Statistics suggest the average is four years, but for some women it can be as long as fifteen years. Signs and symptoms can vary throughout and continue after menopause has occurred. More and more women are experiencing perimenopause in their late thirties and early forties. Some woman in their sixties and seventies still report experiencing hot flushes which aren't attributed to any other cause.

(In this book I will be using menopause to mean the time from when menopausal symptoms are first felt until they cease.)

Menopause is not just about hormones rampaging through your system, sometimes having weird, unsettling and unpredictable effects on you. Research is showing your whole being is rewiring, especially your brain. Hence the forgetfulness and brain fog that many women complain of. This is comparable to puberty. It is puberty in reverse, as once you've entered menopause your hormone levels, if you are fit and healthy, are similar to what they were as a child.

From puberty until menopause your monthly hormone cycle is designed to have you focus on reproduction and nurturing of others. As these hormones start to wane, it can feel unsettling and lead to big changes in your life, not just physically but also emotionally.

This time often corresponds with your children moving out into the world, resulting in what is referred to as 'empty nest syndrome'. Many women also find themselves facing marital separation, divorce, change of career direction and dealing with ageing parents at this time.

What Causes Menopause?

Age is the main cause of the menopause. Women are born with a set number of egg-producing follicles in their ovaries. One egg, or occasionally two, are released each month. This occurs from puberty until menopause, except during pregnancy or because of hormonal imbalance. Anorexia, excessive exercise and stress can cause cessation of a woman's menses, (commonly referred to as a 'period') as they cause hormonal imbalances.

When your follicles run out menopause occurs. This is usually around the age of fifty, but can be as early as thirty-five or as late as sixty. The ovaries don't abruptly stop working but start slowing down. This transition is the perimenopause. Menopause is a natural occurrence except if it is caused by surgical removal of the ovaries, uterus (womb), chemotherapy or pelvic radiation.

The medical profession often say menopausal symptoms are due to insufficient oestrogen. This may be true for a few women, but the majority today are more likely to be oestrogen dominant. Oestrogen dominance causes breast tenderness, weight gain, bloating and mood swings. You are probably familiar with this as it's what you experienced in puberty. It's strange, but doctors will report the ups and downs of puberty as being due to high oestrogen exposure, but the same symptoms during menopause are labelled as oestrogen deficiency!

Watch Kate's Menopausal Story
http://www.pamlob.com/kates-story/

A Simple Biology Lesson

You have three main sex hormones; oestrogen, progesterone and testosterone, that are produced in the adrenal glands and ovaries. After menopause production is mainly in the adrenal glands, which sit on top of your kidneys. These three sex hormones are made from a precursor hormone Dehydroepiandrosterone (DHEA), which is made in the adrenal glands and brain.

From the onset of puberty until menopause, except during pregnancy, it's normal for a woman to go through a monthly menstrual cycle that is between 23 and 35 days on average. The main purpose of each cycle is reproduction. If fertilisation of the egg does not occur, the woman experiences her monthly bleed. This is due to the elimination of the womb lining that developed in the second half of her cycle, ready to receive the egg if it became fertilised by a sperm.

During each monthly cycle, a variety of hormones release at different times to stimulate the release of the egg and to prepare the womb for a fertilised egg and if this doesn't occur to shed the womb lining. There is no need to get booged down trying to understand all the hormones and how they work as the only ones important to understand for menopause are oestrogen, progesterone and testosterone.

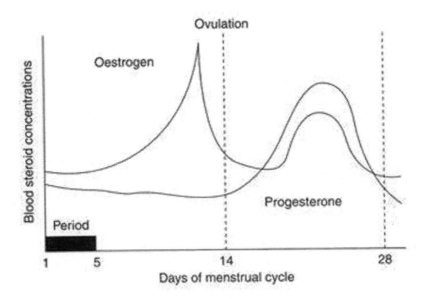

In the first part of the menstrual cycle, starting on day one of menstruation, known as the follicular phase, large amounts of oestrogen are produced by the ovaries, to prepare the follicles for release of an egg. It is this period that varies the most from woman to woman, or cycle to cycle.

At about day 14 of a 28-day cycle, ovulation occurs and the egg is released into the fallopian tubes ready to be fertilised by a male sperm within the next 24 hours. At this time levels of oestrogen begin to fall and progesterone begins to rise, to build up the lining of the womb in preparation for a fertilised egg. This is known as the luteal phase and this is the time when women experience bloating, breast tenderness, lethargy, depression and irritability, often referred to as pre-menstrual tension (PMT).

The cause of PMT is unknown, but it is likely to be due to the levels of the different hormones that get released during this part of the cycle. Studies suggest that it is oestrogen that causes the bloating and breast tenderness and other studies suggest it's how some women metabolise progesterone. PMT becomes more common in women as they enter the perimenopause.

If fertilisation has not taken place at around day 26-28 progesterone and oestrogen levels drop significantly and menstruation occurs.

As women approach menopause, the length of their menstrual cycle can vary. For some women the length of each cycle increases and for others it shortens, or there can be swings from one to the other.

It has also been discovered women don't necessarily ovulate in every cycle and the likelihood of anovulatory (egg less) cycles increases with age. In this type of cycle, progesterone is very low, or not produced at all, with potential devastating effects on fertility and increasing the risk of osteoporosis, breast cancer, fibroids and endometriosis.

Effects of Progesterone and Oestrogen

Your hormones are an essential part of your physiology. Without them you wouldn't survive. They are something you take for granted until they go array. The system that controls your hormones is called the endocrine system and is incredibly complicated and still not fully understood.

To complicate things further, hormone levels are notoriously difficult to measure. Just thinking about them or walking into a doctor's office can make huge differences in their levels. The most accurate way to measure them is with a 24-hour urine collection.

Effects of Oestrogen	Effects of Progesterone
Develops and releases the egg	Maintains lining of the uterus
Increases blood clotting	Normalises blood clotting
Increases risk of breast cancer	Protects against breast cancer

Thins skin	Strengthens skin
Encourages water and salt retention	Is a natural diuretic
Increases the lining of the uterus	Helps maintain a pregnancy
Lays down fat stores	Encourages the use of stored energy and burning of fat
Can cause headaches	Is a precursor to important stress hormones
Can cause depression	Anti-depressant
Decreases libido	Increases libido
Slows down reabsorption of bone	Stimulates the building of new bone

Oestrogen and progesterone seem to have opposing functions, but their actions are interrelated. "Progesterone tends to balance out many of the negative side effects of oestrogen and at the same time can't function properly in the body without the help of oestrogen," (Lee 2004).

Research shows that for many women at the time of menopause, progesterone levels are falling proportionately faster than levels of oestrogen and in some cases, are lower than in men. This is despite the fact that oestrogen, like all the steroid hormones within the body, derives from progesterone.

When oestrogen is dominant, the following symptoms are likely:

* Acceleration of ageing

- Allergies

- Anxiety

- Autoimmune disorders

- Breast tenderness

- Breast, uterine cancer

- Decreased sex drive

- Depression

- Weight Gain

- Fatigue

- Fibroids

- Gallbladder disease

- Craving for caffeine and sweets

- Hair loss

- Headaches

- Irritability

- Memory Loss

- Water retention

- Insomnia

- Osteoporosis

- Thyroid dysfunction

- Stroke.

Oestrogen dominance occurs because of stress, diet, toxin overload and lifestyle.

The Role of Testosterone

Testosterone is often thought of as the male hormone. However, testosterone is equally important to women, it's just in lower quantities. Testosterone is needed to build muscle mass, maintain bone density, maintain a healthy weight, libido and creativity.

Your testosterone levels may be low if you experience:

- Insomnia

- Vaginal dryness

- Loss of sex drive

- Fatigue

- Weight gain around your middle.

Testosterone can dip:

- At the beginning of perimenopause

- If you come off the contraceptive pill

- After removal of the ovaries

- If your progesterone is low

- If you are stressed.

Testosterone levels can be maintained by eating saturated fats, especially avocado, increasing your intake of zinc by eating seeds and beans, exercising and reducing stress, or taking a supplement prescribed by your doctor.

Signs of Menopausal Transition

The transition into menopause can vary enormously. Some women experience none or few symptoms other than their periods become irregular until they stop altogether. Others experience horrendous problems that leave them barely able to function.

The symptoms that women experience are not just due to hormone imbalances. Health, lifestyle, culture and expectation also play a big part.

Women the world over will have similar hormone changes if everything is working normally as they go through menopause. But not all women around the world, or from previous generations, have the same signs and symptoms.

Research shows that Chinese and Japanese woman rarely report issues with hot flushes and night sweats whereas three quarters of Caucasian woman will report this symptom and the percentage is even higher for African Americans.

From my own experience and research, I believe the main causes of menopausal symptoms today in the western world are:

- Stress

- Lifestyle (including diet)

- Beliefs

- Toxins

- Disconnection from the whole of you and especially your feminine essence.

I will be looking at each of these in detail in further chapters.

Common Menopausal Symptoms

- Time between periods gets longer or shorter

- Heavy, cramping periods

- Very light periods

- Fluctuating period length

- Hot flushes

- Night sweats

- Skin becomes thinner and drier especially in vagina and urinary tract

- Mood swings

- Irritability

- Anxiety

- Panic attacks

- Sleep problems

- Changes in libido

- Joint pain

- Memory problems

- Frequent urination or incontinence.

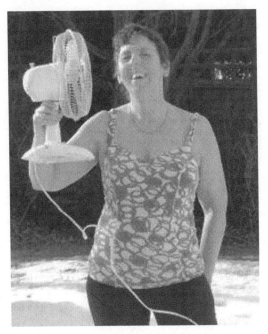

Have you noticed how alike these symptoms are to oestrogen dominance?

All of these symptoms can also be attributed to stress. For example, hot flushes and night sweats may result from stress and is why they are being reported by women in their twenties, sixties and seventies.

Stress leads to raised cortisol levels that effect all your other hormone levels. Decreasing the stress in your life could ensure a graceful and easy menopause transition. I believe the most likely reason why you are experiencing menopausal difficulties is because you are stressed. I will be looking at stress in detail in the next chapter.

Menopause Treatments

Many women want an instant fix, a magic pill that will cure them instantly with no side effects. Sorry to disillusion you, but the truth is there is no magic treatment. Your body has an amazing capacity to maintain balance and heal itself if you treat it right.

Getting rid of your menopausal symptoms, plus stepping onto the road of feeling and looking good well into old age, occurs when you decide that what you are doing right now is not working and it's time to change.

Every one of us is unique, so exactly what needs to change and how quickly you get results varies from person to person.

Change only happens when you start taking action and the first action is to accept what is happening right now is not working.

Remember...

'WHAT YOU RESIST PERSISTS'

Habits take twenty-one to ninety days on average to change and I'm here to support and guide you on this journey.

To lead a happy, healthy, joyful rest of your life without risks from medication, diet and lifestyle changes are required. Later in the book I will share with you some amazing practices and strategies to transform your life. First, a little on the more standard treatments that are available, to help you make an informed decision on what is right for you.

Many of the treatments available from pharmaceutical drugs don't deal with the cause of your symptoms, so are little better than a sticking plaster covering a wound. They can be helpful in the short term to reduce the pain and discomfort you are experiencing. However they all have potential side effects, or cause adverse reactions, especially if you take other medications, including contraceptives.

In its drive to manufacture patent drugs that it can charge high prices for, the pharmaceutical industry strives to separate an active ingredient from a plant and make a synthetic substance not found in nature. In doing so, it frequently results in there being harmful side effects and the body is often unable to eliminate them effectively.

If used properly and in the correct doses, plant medicines, such as herbal remedies, rarely have any negative effects. Your body has evolved over time and has adapted to interact with natural substances you ingest, to help repair and maintain energy. Anything you don't need is eliminated via the digestive tract, liver or kidneys.

Herbs may be natural, but they can also be toxic if not taken correctly, or in combination with prescription medicine. Always check with a pharmacist before using any herbal or vitamin supplement if you are taking medication. Working with a herbalist or naturopath is advisable as they can give you advice on what is best for you.

Watch Jocelyn's Menopause Story
http://www.pamlob.com/jocelyns-story

Hormone Replacement Therapy

The one treatment that many women turn to and most doctors recommend, is Hormone Replacement Therapy (HRT). This is due to the belief that women at the time of menopause are deficient in oestrogen. By giving women hormone replacements, doctors believe it will stop hot flushes, give them energy and the elixir of youth.

In fact, most women today are oestrogen dominant and it is the lack of balancing progesterone that is the problem. Even though most HRT today contains progesterone, it is in an artificial form which the body cannot synthesise effectively. Many doctors believe synthetic progesterone is identical to natural progesterone, though research has shown this is not true. Unfortunately, doctors rarely have time to keep up-to-date with all the research. They rely heavily on the information from drug reps and the pharmaceutical industry, who are only interested in selling their products.

Doctors often persuade women to take HRT in the belief that they are protecting themselves from heart disease and osteoporosis. This was why I agreed to take it, believing I was at significant risk as I turned menopausal at forty. However, no large clinical trial has shown taking HRT has a significant effect in reducing your risk of heart disease or osteoporosis. Wish I had known this when I had my hysterectomy and was persuaded to take HRT!

Whilst my husband was ill, my feelings of exhaustion increased, so I upped my HRT dose for a while in the belief it would give me more energy. I quickly realised it was making me feel worse, not just on the energy front, but brain fog and hot flushes increased and I went back to the original dose. When I came off HRT completely a year later, my health improved rapidly.

At the turn of the 21st century, The Women's Health Initiative did a long-term study looking at the health of 16,000 women aged fifty to seventy-nine years. One of the things the study examined was the side effects of the most commonly prescribed HRT drug at the time, 'PremPro'. This drug combines Premarin, an oestrogen taken from horse urine and Provera, a synthetic progesterone.

In 2002, three years into its five-year programme, the study was stopped as it had shown women using PremPro, "had a 29 percent higher risk of breast cancer, a 26 percent higher risk of heart disease and a 41 percent higher risk of stroke," (Dr Lee, 2004). This led to many women at the time stopping their HRT, or changing to a different brand. Despite this research, PremPro is still regularly prescribed today and many doctors are unaware of this study.

A study conducted by Oxford University for the Cochrane Library, published in March 2015, showed HRT had no effect on reducing heart disease and increased the risk of stroke, blood clots and slightly raised the risk of ovarian cancer. The researchers concluded their results "provide strong evidence that treatment with hormone therapy in post-menopausal women overall … has little if any benefit and causes an increase in the risk of stroke and venous thromboembolic events."

Possible Side Effects of HRT

- Weight gain

- Bloating

- Nausea

- Breast tenderness

- Breakthrough bleeding

- Leg cramps

- Headaches

- Indigestion.

Increased risk of:

- Blood clots

- Deep vein thrombosis

- Pulmonary embolism

- Breast cancer

- Cancer of the uterus

- Ovarian Cancer

- Heart Disease

- Stroke.

HRT may be beneficial in the short term following a hysterectomy that includes removal of the ovaries, whilst a woman is still menstruating. This allows her body time to adjust to the sudden loss of oestrogen and progesterone previously produced by the ovaries. However, if you are not stressed and your adrenals are working normally, then the adjustment should happen quite quickly.

If you don't address the cause of your menopausal symptoms, at best HRT will simply delay the experience of the symptoms. You are merely slowing down the inevitable!

Anti-Depressants

Even more frightening than the number of women given HRT, is the number being prescribed anti-depressants for menopausal symptoms such as hot flushes, even when they have no symptoms of depression.

Research into anti-depressants has found they are no more effective than a placebo in mild-to-moderate depression. They came to be used for menopausal symptoms because the initial trials by the pharmaceutical industry reported participants being relieved of their hot flushes. However, no baseline data for the number of hot flushes participants were having was connected before the trials, making the results worthless.

Anti-depressants are addictive and have side effects including fatigue, irritability, anxiety, trouble sleeping and loss of sexual desire. They can also disconnect you from your emotions. You might be pleased not to feel sadness and negativity, but do you not wish to feel joy and happiness? We need all of our emotions to function as healthy human beings, just as a rainbow needs each of its colours to be a rainbow.

Bio-identical Hormones

Bio-identical hormones are derived from plants and are made in a laboratory. They have an identical molecular structure to hormones produced by the human body. In contrast, the hormones in HRT are synthetic and though their structure is similar to your natural hormones, they are not a perfect fit to your hormone receptor cells. This incapability causes the side effects. Therefore, as bio-identical hormones can connect with the hormone receptor cells, side effects shouldn't occur. However, bio-identical hormones cannot be patented, so there are few scientific studies on their effectiveness or side effects.

To be prescribed bio-identical hormones you need to see a doctor who specialises in them. They will first take blood and saliva tests to determine your hormone levels. A prescription is then made up of oestrogen, progesterone, testosterone and DHEA to meet your individual needs. Your levels will then be monitored and appropriate dosage adjustments made.

Natural Progesterone

An alternative to HRT available without prescription is natural progesterone cream made from wild yam or soy. (Be aware that not all wild yam extracts contain progesterone, so choose a product that has natural progesterone cream on the label). The body utilises and processes this cream in the same way as it uses progesterone produced by the body, so there are no side effects. Research has shown progesterone in this form is very helpful in reversing osteoporosis.

In 1999, a double-blind study of progesterone cream conducted by Helene Leonetti MD showed that 83% of women in the progesterone cream group experienced relief from their menopausal symptoms versus only 19% in the control group (Lee, 2004).

Some doctors will prescribe progesterone cream, but make sure that it is natural and not synthetic. It is available without prescription but I would advise you to see a naturopathic doctor who can check your personal needs.

During his lifetime Dr. Lee became a leading light in the use of natural progesterone cream. His book 'What Your Doctor May Not Tell You About Menopause' recommends using, "a two ounce container of progesterone cream that contains 900 to 1,000 mg of progesterone (a 1.6 to 2.0 percent progesterone cream). This amounts to about 40 mg per ½ teaspoon, 20 mg per ¼ teaspoon, and 10 mg per ⅛ teaspoon."

The dose he recommends for menopausal women is 10 to 12mg, or ⅛ teaspoon of progesterone cream per day for 25 days of the month. The cream is best applied twice daily, with a larger proportion of the dose at bedtime to areas where your skin is thinner such as chest, inner arms, neck and face. It is good practice to alternate the areas of application. If you are still menstruating, Dr. Lee suggests 15 to 20 mg of progesterone cream daily in the 2 weeks prior to your period.

In a three-year trial Dr. Lee researched the effects of natural progesterone on his own patients aged 38-83 who were using the cream. His patients reported not only relief from menopausal symptoms, but also relief from "a wide array of other symptoms as diverse as dry eyes, bloating, irritability, gall bladder problems, osteoporosis pain, hair loss, and lumpy or sore breasts," (Lee, 2004).

From observing these results, Dr. Lee started to include bone density measurements to monitor osteoporosis and found there was significant improvement in all his patients.

Power of Plants

There are many different herbal remedies available, in tablet or tincture format, as individual ingredients or as a combination. When combined together they have a synergetic effect, which is greater than taking the herbs individually. I found tinctures were the most effective. Choose ones which are organic, to avoid overloading your liver further with pesticides that may be on the herbs. Buy reputable brands as there are a lot of cheap poor quality products available.

Even though herbs are natural, it is still possible to overdose, or have an intolerance or allergic reaction. Always take in the lowest dose possible initially and check with a pharmacist to ensure that none of the ingredients will react with any other medication you may be taking.

Sage

Sage is a herb you may have growing in your garden. It can be used in cooking, or as a tea, but it is also available in tablet form or as a tincture.

It is useful in helping with hot flushes and night sweats.

Black Cohosh

Black cohosh is a herb related to the buttercup family and acts as a selective oestrogen receptor modulator. It can stimulate oestrogen receptors appropriately in some parts of the body and not in others, whereas HRT merely replaces hormones.

It is available as a tea, tincture or tablet.

It is useful in helping with hot flushes, night sweats, depression, anxiety and irritability.

Agnus Castus

Agnus castus is a herb from the Mediterranean classified as an adaptogen. It has a balancing effect on your hormones, increasing them if they are too low, or decreasing if they are too high.

It is good for mood swings, tension, PMS, anxiety and breast tenderness.

Milk Thistle

Milk thistle helps improve liver function. One of the roles of the liver is to detoxify your body of unwanted substances. In this day and age, with the toxic overload from our environment, the liver needs plenty of support.

Dong Quai

Dong quai is also referred to as female ginseng. It's a herb used in Traditional Chinese Medicine to help with hot flushes, night sweats, fatigue and sleep disturbance. It also strengthens bones so is good for Osteoporosis and can have a blood sugar lowering effect. It's available as a capsule, tea or tincture.

Red Clover

Red clover has natural levels of oestrogen and contains high amounts of nutrients such as potassium, thiamine, calcium, chromium, magnesium, niacin, phosphorus and vitamin C.

It is effective in the treatment of hot flushes, night sweats, insomnia, premenstrual syndrome, plus headaches and cramps associated with the menstrual cycle.

Maca

Maca grows in the high plateaus of the Andes in Peru. It has been cultivated as a vegetable crop for over 3000 years. Its root is used for medicine. It's available as a powder that can be added to food, or in tablet form.

Maca helps improve energy, stamina, hormonal balance, memory and boosts the immune system.

Ginkgo Biloba

Ginkgo biloba is a herb from the Chinese maidenhair tree. It has been found to have a rejuvenating effect on the brain. Research has shown it improves memory, concentration and learning ability.

WARNING Ginkgo biloba should not be taken with HRT, the contraceptive pill, fertility drugs or other hormonal treatments. It may also interact with anti-inflammatory drugs such as Ibuprofen. If you are on any medication, check with your pharmacist or doctor before using.

St John's Wort

Research has found St John's Wort is more effective than anti-depressants in treating mild-to-moderate depression. It is also antibacterial, antioxidant and anti-inflammatory.

WARNING It can react with, or make some prescription medicines, including contraceptives, ineffective, so you **must check** with your pharmacist or doctor before taking.

Watch Elizabeth's Menopause Story
http://www.pamlob.com/elizabeths-story

Ladycare Device

The Ladycare device is a magnet type device that you attach to your underwear in the pelvic area. It is believed it works by balancing the sympathetic and parasympathetic parts of the autonomic nervous system. Research suggests over 70% of users experience a significant reduction in hot sweats after a month of use. This product may be less effective if you are stressed.

Osteoporosis

Osteoporosis is often blamed on menopause and is often cited as one of the major reasons to go on HRT. It was certainly the reason I did. My research has pulled up a number of myths on osteoporosis and I want to share them with you, so you can make an informed decision on the best way to protect your bone health.

Osteoporosis is a disease in which the mesh-like structure within your bones becomes thin, increasing the risk of fractures from minor bumps or falls. Though it can affect all bones of your body, the most commonly affected bones are wrists, hips and spine.

Myth 1

Osteoporosis is a disease of menopausal women and it is an oestrogen deficiency disease.

Though it occurs more frequently in women, it also affects men. It is more common in men low in testosterone and women who are low in progesterone.

Myth 2

Osteoporosis is treatable by drinking loads of milk and taking calcium supplements.

Both in fact, make osteoporosis worse. In countries with a much lower intake of calcium, there is a lower incidence of the disease.

Myth 3

Bone mass declines as a normal consequence of ageing.

Examination of ancient bones has found no significant bone loss at any age.

Today when women reach perimenopause, many may have already lost 20-30 percent of their bone mass.

Bone cells are normally constantly being regenerated and broken down, this is what allows a fracture to heal whatever your age. In fact, your skeleton is replaced about every seven years. It is one of the roles of oestrogen post-puberty to control the rate old bone is being broken down and progesterone helps to build new bone. The two hormones should work in harmony, but if there is more oestrogen than progesterone, there is less new bone production and osteoporosis occurs.

Myth 4

HRT will prevent osteoporosis.

Researchers in the 1970s discovered that HRT slightly decreased the rate of bone loss. Large pharmaceutical companies leapt on this fact as a way of promoting HRT and their statements have led to the belief that osteoporosis is due to oestrogen deficiency.

When this research is looked at closely, the population of women examined was too small to be significant and the measurement of bone mass levels was imprecise. Nor did it take into account that the HRT also contained progesterone. Also note that the research says "decreased the rate of bone loss," thus oestrogen does not help in replacing bone already lost.

Prevention/ Treatment

- Weight-bearing exercise
- Minimum intake of processed table salt (use sea salt or Himalayan rock salt instead)
- Maintain a normal weight for your height
- Eat plenty of vegetables
- Magnesium
- Sunlight
- Vitamin D3
- Vitamin K
- Boron
- Strontium
- Natural progesterone cream.

Research has shown that women who are slim, vegetarian, who exercise and do not take regular prescribed medication are less likely to suffer from osteoporosis than women who eat meat daily, rarely exercise and regularly take prescribed medication.

CHAPTER 2

Are You Addicted to Stress?

"I promise you nothing is as chaotic as it seems. Nothing is worth diminishing your health. Nothing is worth poisoning yourself into stress, anxiety, and fear."

Steve Maraboli

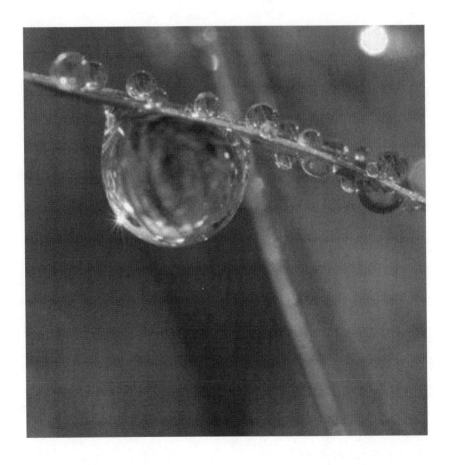

ARE YOU ADDICTED TO STRESS?

Watch Are You Addicted to Stress
http://www.pamlob.com/are-you-addicted-to-stress/

Stress is the number one cause of hormone imbalance and I believe the main reason why so many women today experience symptoms blamed on menopause.

There is a saying, "life begins at forty." For a lot of woman in years gone by, as they hit their forties, life in many ways was getting easier as the hard grind of getting on the career ladder, building relationships, setting up home and starting a family was behind them. This is not the case for many women today.

Today…

- It's more common for women to be just starting a family in their late thirties and early forties.

- The majority of women are juggling work and childcare, as a dual income is required to pay the bills and have a few luxuries.

- Divorce statistics are on the rise, leaving many women responsible for the family income and majority, if not all the childcare.

- A lifelong career with the same employer is becoming rare and an expectation of working long hours and meeting endless, often ridiculous targets is making work life much more stressful.

What is Stress?

"Suffering becomes beautiful when anyone bears great calamities with cheerfulness, not through insensibility but through greatness of mind."
Aristotle

Stress is a mental and physical response to the challenges and demands you experience in life. It is not a disease, but dis-ease as it is something you create in your own mind. Thus stress means something different to everyone. What will be stressful to one person can be motivating to another.

You have a choice whether to be stressed or not.

A small amount of stress can be good for you as it can be a great motivator and can improve performance. Acute stress occurs from having to flee from a burning building, or meet a tight deadline at work. This can be good for you and may even save your life. However, if stress comes from a place of not having enough time, money, skill, or energy on a daily basis, this is chronic stress and it threatens your health and stops you fulfilling your goals and achieving your dreams.

Chronic stress does not just come from external sources, but also from not having the right nutrients in your diet, not getting enough exercise, having the wrong climate, or the wrong work or home environment for your body's unique needs. Some people can cope with clutter, or an environment that is too hot or too cold, whilst for others they need everything to be organised, minimalist and quiet.

Another stressor is living life from your head space, feeling guilty about the past and worried about the future, rather than being in the 'now,' connected with your body, emotions, energy, feminine essence and intuition.

Chronic stress decreases performance and leads to health issues including heart disease, cancer, depression, relationship breakdowns and employment problems.

Chronic stress keeps you living in a pond. Living in the 'River of Life' doesn't mean you won't experience stressful events, but they will be just that, events, which may be fun or not, which will pass as you move on down the river!

Stress is a response evolved thousands of years ago to keep you safe. Faced with a predator such as a lion, you had the choice to run away or stand and fight. Once the lion was out of sight and you were safely back with your tribe, you relaxed and the stress hormones left the body.

However today…

- Numerous people, and you may be one of them, are acting as if the lion is constantly in your home, or office! Is he behind you, or lurking under your desk?

- You may have created a long 'To Do' list that, despite your best efforts, only seems to grow.

- You feel overwhelmed as you rush from one thing to another and try to do several things at once.

- Many people have demands on your time and attention. You are exhausted and irritated just trying desperately to keep up.

By not creating space and time for relaxation, the stress hormones never leave your body. Over time your body, mind and emotions experience the symptoms of chronic stress.

Chronic stress occurs when the body is constantly under the influence of the stress hormones:

- Adrenaline

- Norepinephrine

- Cortisol.

These hormones unbalance your nervous system. The sympathetic nervous system that readies you for 'fight or flight' starts to dominate and slows down the functions of the parasympathetic nervous system. The parasympathetic nervous system is responsible for helping you digest your food, rest, sleep and heal. These are unimportant when your life is on the line running from a lion, but to maintain health and wellbeing, they are essential.

Regular, or permanently raised levels of these stress hormones, especially cortisol, and the dumbing down of the parasympathetic nervous system, are a causal factor in most serious health issues, including heart disease and cancer. They are also a significant contributor to raised blood pressure and blood glucose levels, obesity, suppression of the immune system and yes, menopausal symptoms.

They can exacerbate existing health issues such as asthma, arthritis and skin conditions. They may also make you look older than you are as they can cause skin to become dry and more wrinkled. They can also adversely affect your relationships and employment due to fatigue, being short tempered, forgetful, tearful or agitated.

Stress is cumulative. I often describe stress as a set of children's building blocks, stacked one upon another. It might only be the addition of a small brick that sets the tower swaying, or leads to collapse. Often it is the small, everyday niggles that have more effect than the big ones.

It is often said the way to deal with your problems is to experience a major problem as it puts all the niggling little ones into perspective.

Stress comes from external events such as:

- Moving house

- Getting married

- Redundancy or retirement

- Bereavement

- Divorce

- Holidays and family celebrations

- Illness or injury

- Financial difficulties

- Change and uncertainty

- Trying to balance work and family needs

- A large 'To Do' List.

Stress also comes from internal dialogues:

- Negative thoughts

- Guilt

- Judgments

- Negative beliefs about yourself

- Worry about the future

- Placing too much pressure on yourself, through high expectations and perfectionism.

- Disconnection from your body, emotions, energy and intuition.

- Disconnection from your feminine essence.

An often overlooked reason for stress is that society today teaches you logic and scientific reasoning are the only ways to think, behave and be successful. This leads to imbalance, as you are only listening to the limited beliefs and perceptions of your mind as programmed by the media, culture and upbringing, and not the intuitive guidance from your heart. More on this later.

Are you Addicted to Stress?

Do you start your day worrying you don't have enough time, enough energy or enough resources to achieve everything on your 'To Do' list? This immediately puts the brain into a state of stress before you've even gotten out of bed!

Stress not only affects your stress hormones, it also has a negative effect on nearly all of your hormones. Kirsten Sweeting Morreli, founder of the Red Tent Revival, suggests that stress is the 'New Crack' as so many people are addicted to it.

As with many other addictions, many of you will be 'in denial.' For many women, stress is the unmentioned elephant in the room.

Stress is an insidious, quiet disorder that for many has become embedded in their tissues and psyche. An accepted norm which in reality is far from what normal should be.

When you are addicted to stress your cortisol levels are constantly imbalanced. Cortisol, as well as being part of your stress response, is also responsible for controlling blood sugar, blood pressure and the immune system. Therefore, if it is out of balance your whole system is out of balance too and disease becomes a higher and higher risk.

How do You Become Addicted to Stress?

A spike in cortisol and adrenaline gives you the power and drive to 'fight or flight' when faced with danger, or when you experience fear from public speaking, jumping from an airplane, or doing something new for the first time. It can give you a buzz and the ability to boost your performance.

Some actors say the day they stop feeling fearful and nervous before going on stage is the day to retire from acting, as they will no longer be giving their best. This is good stress as it gives power, passion and motivation for a short duration.

However, chronic stress and anxiety causes cortisol and adrenaline levels to be permanently high. If you are regularly anxious or stressed, your body gets used to a higher level of cortisol and adrenaline. In turn you need ever increasing amounts to feel alive, to get the buzz and the drive that being under pressure can give you. Therefore, you seek out conflict in order to feel the high that adrenaline and cortisol provides, raising your base level even higher.

Many people today have long 'To Do' lists. Women who are working and juggling the needs of home and kids are especially prone. They rush their kids from one after school activity to another, cook, do the housework and end up subconsciously competing with other mums to see who can do the most.

Gynaecologist, Dr. Sara Gottfried, refers to this as the 'Mum Martyr Club,' and you don't have to be a mum to be a member. Anyone who is mothering someone (it could be being at the beck and call of your boss) can join. You are a member of this club if you feel like you are pushing a huge rock uphill each day to stay on top of everything that needs to be done.

Men are physically and mentally wired to push rocks up hill and may be happy to do so all day long, but women are not. It strains the female body even more, leading to even higher cortisol levels. A vicious cycle ensues.

Signs and Symptoms of Stress Addiction

- You get a second wind late at night and believe you are being really creative and getting loads done.

- You can't lose weight despite eating healthily throughout the day. When stressed you build belly fat four times faster than elsewhere in your body.

- You come home and need a glass or two of wine to destress. This doesn't really help, as alcohol actually increases cortisol levels.

- You have a tiredness dip sometime between 2-5pm when all you want to do is take a nap.

- You often feel tired but wired.

- You have difficulty in winding down before going to sleep.

- You are addicted to having drama and conflict in your life.

- You have low blood pressure, so feel dizzy if you get up too quickly.

- You find yoga and meditation doesn't help you relax. (Stillness helps men relax but often doesn't work for women).

- You carry a lot of resentment.

If you said yes to three or more of the above list, I'm sorry to say, you are addicted to stress and it's time to be aware and accept this fact.

Awareness is the first action in being able to do something about it, followed by acceptance. Acceptance does not mean you have to like it, rather it's just about acknowledging and not resisting it. When you are in denial or in resistance, nothing changes.

Stress often makes it difficult for you to prioritise what is most important to you. Having too much choice can make you even more stressed and likely to accept whatever comes along.

Take some time (you deserve a break) and take a look at each area of your life:

- *Work*
- *Home*
- *Money*
- *Relationships*
- *Health*
- *Recreation.*

Assess what is most important to you?

Do you achieve a balance in all these areas?

Which areas are giving you the most stress?

Devoting all your time to only one or two areas will increase your stress.

Clarify your major priorities and goals to achieve more balance and less stress in your life. Break these down into smaller and smaller manageable action steps, then start taking SMALL steps to achieve what you want.

DOWNLOAD Playbook-Are You Addicted to
Stress?
http://www.pamlob.com/are-you-addicted-to-stress-
playbook1

A Simple Science Lesson on Stress

I believe having a basic understanding of how your body works can
help you understand what is wrong. It puts you in a better position to
ask the right questions of your healthcare professionals, who
frequently don't have all the answers.

You are the expert on your own body and health.

Yes, I am skeptical of doctors, in terms of them knowing what is wrong
with me, or offering the right treatment for me. It took twenty years
for me to get a medical diagnosis of endometriosis and it was my
reflexologist who first identified it!

I trained as a nurse, therefore I'm familiar with the medical model of
health. I see its biggest failing is its focus on signs and symptoms and
not the cause of disease. It also does not recognise each one of us is
an individual with a unique life and needs. Doctors unfortunately are
usually pushed for time and for ease, they reach for the prescription
pad. They are excellent in a medical emergency, but struggle when it
comes to long-term health issues. Very few have any training in
nutrition, preventative and holistic health, or alternative and
complementary therapies.

Your Hormones and Stress

Stress is a natural response to keep us safe. When you are faced with
danger of any kind, a lion hiding in the tall grass, an accident, or
being shouted at by your boss, your lower brain (often referred to as
the reptilian brain) takes over from your thinking brain, which cannot
respond fast enough to 'fight or flight.' It sends a message to your
adrenals to give you a surge of adrenaline and cortisol to raise your
blood pressure. More oxygen is then sent to your brain and for

glucose to be released into your muscles, to give you the strength to run, find help, or deal with the situation.

Once the situation is over, cortisol levels return to normal, but today's addiction to stress means that the cortisol boost rarely or never gets turned off. This results in your lower brain being permanently vigilant, looking for threats from your relationships with your partner, boss, within your emails and 'To Do' list. This leads to the symptoms often blamed on menopause of poor sleep, additional belly fat and anxiety.

Your hormones are an essential part of your physiology. Without them you wouldn't survive, but they are something you take for granted until they go array. Your endocrine system controls your hormones and is incredibly complicated and still not fully understood.

An added complication is that hormone levels are notoriously difficult to measure. Just thinking about them or walking into a doctor's office can make huge differences. Chronic stress has a major impact on all hormone levels.

The Role of Adrenal Glands

Your adrenal glands are small glands that sit on top of your kidneys. They produce cortisol, adrenaline, noradrenaline, aldosterone and your sex hormones of testosterone, progesterone and oestrogen. They are made up of two parts, the inner medulla and the outer cortex.

Your adrenal glands play a big part in your stress response.

The medulla helps regulate your sympathetic nervous system, whose primary role is to stimulate your body's fight-or-flight stress response by secreting two hormones, adrenaline and noradrenaline. They raise your blood pressure and blood sugar, so you have the energy to run, or stand and fight.

When your body is under the influence of adrenaline, you tend to be very alert, focused and energised. This state is much admired in the business world and so people keep wanting to feel this high. To reproduce it, they have learnt by being angry or fearful they can get the high that they are looking for. Fear and anger are common bedfellows of stress. The bad news is that adrenaline should not be used long-term, only short-term and in an emergency. Overusing it will eventually exhaust the adrenal medulla.

At the time of menopause, the adrenal glands take over most of the production of oestrogen and progesterone from the ovaries. Yet if they are busy producing cortisol and adrenaline, they don't have the capacity to produce progesterone and oestrogen as well. Therefore, along come the hot flushes, night sweats, poor sleep, low libido, moodiness and foggy thinking. These are also symptoms of stress for both men and women in any age group.

It is most likely stress and not menopause that is causing most, if not all, of the symptoms blamed on menopause.

The Role of Cortisol

Cortisol is often referred to as the stress hormone, but it is so much more.

Cortisol's main role is to increase glucose levels in your blood and store excess in your liver, so you have enough energy to keep you alive. It is responsible for stimulating the liver to remove toxins, aid digestion and reduce inflammation, whilst controlling hunger cravings, sleep patterns, physical activity and capacity to deal with stress.

Your cortisol levels are designed to differ throughout the day. They are high in the morning to give you energy to get up and get going. They then reduce gradually during the day and are at a minimum level at bedtime, so you are able to drift off to sleep. When your cortisol level is at its lowest around midnight, your body's cells can repair and heal.

However, when your system is constantly stressed your cortisol levels stay high, making it difficult to fall asleep at night. Thus your cells don't have the opportunity to repair and heal sufficiently, increasing your risk of illness. It can also result in you having low cortisol in the morning, so you wake feeling tired and find it difficult to get going.

The action of all your hormones is interrelated. If your cortisol levels are following a normal pattern of being high in the morning and low in the evening, your melatonin levels (which respond to light and dark) act in reverse, helping you to sleep. Melatonin also has a major role in controlling the rhythm of your body temperature.

If your cortisol levels are constantly high, your body's hormone receptors start becoming resistant, so you require more of each hormone to feel their effect. When none, or few of your hormones are working optimally, you can feel rotten.

High cortisol also causes the brain to be less sensitive to oestrogen. This is why it can appear that a woman is oestrogen deficient and getting hot flushes, when if tested, her oestrogen levels are normal or high. If supplementary oestrogen is given in the form of HRT, you are likely to experience weight gain, water retention and moodiness and unfortunately still have hot flushes. Whilst cortisol remains high, nothing will really change, apart from the possibility of adding more symptoms.

As your endocrine system is so finely balanced, adding hormone replacement therapy (even with bio identical hormones) can cause upset rather than balance. It's not possible for drugs to do the fine balancing that happens naturally within your body, minute by minute. Adding a large dose of one hormone imbalances everything else. You might not even be low in oestrogen or progesterone!

I never once in all the years I had treatment for endometriosis, or the five years that I reluctantly took HRT, had my hormone levels tested. I used to laughingly say that I was allergic to my own hormones. Allergic is possibly a bit strong, but I do now believe that I am intolerant to high levels of oestrogen and if I allow stress to creep back into my life, the hot flushes return.

To reduce your menopausal symptoms and to lead a joyful and healthy life, it is vital that you address your levels of stress. You will notice as you read the rest of this book that cortisol, the stress hormone, crops up in every chapter. So you definitely want to stop it running you.

The final chapter of this book gives you lots of tips and strategies that are excellent in reducing stress, but to get you started straight away, try this:

First thing in the morning nourish your brain with something positive.

- *Don't start your day watching the news, or checking emails.*

- *Review what you are grateful for.*

- *Read or listen to something inspirational.*

- *Get out in nature.*

Throughout your day set a timer to alert you every 40-60 minutes, then take a couple of minutes to pause and get up from your desk and do something uplifting.

If you are struggling to identify your stresses and need help in formulating an action plan for your specific needs, or you want support and guidance on your journey, please contact me:

http://www.pamlob.com/contact

CHAPTER 3

You Are What You Eat!

"A positive sense of wellbeing and plenty of energy available whenever needed is what should be regarded as optimum health. That's real vitality."

Prof. Keith Scott-Mumby MB ChB, MD, PhD.

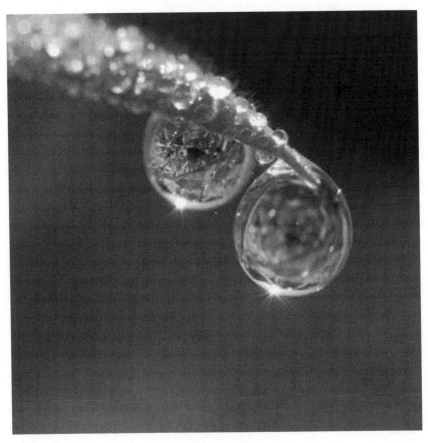

YOU ARE WHAT YOU EAT!

WATCH You are what you Eat!
http://www.pamlob.com/you-are-what-you-eat/

"You are what you eat!" This includes not just the food and drink you put into your mouth, but also what you breathe in through your mouth and nose or absorb through your skin.

Unfortunately, in this modern age, the air we breathe in contains petrochemicals from car exhausts and various toxins from manufacturing processes, crop spraying and power production. Through your skin you absorb toxins from the environment, as well as from cleaning, beauty and skin care products.

I've read somewhere an average western woman absorbs 5lbs (2.27kg) of chemicals into her body every year from make-up and skin care products. Frightening!!

Just take some time to look at some of the labels on your foods and beauty and cleaning products. There will be many ingredients with names you can barely pronounce, let alone know what they actually are and do! Then there are those that aren't mentioned on the label, such as flame-retardants on your clothing and home furnishings, as well as pesticides, herbicides and fungicides on your food and clothing made from natural materials.

The fresh food you eat is frequently covered in pesticides, herbicides and fungicides. Meat and dairy products can contain artificial growth hormones and antibiotics. The water you drink is full of chemicals to kill microorganisms and bacteria in order to make it fit to drink. It can also contain toxic metal salts, pesticides, hormones and depending where you live, fluoride.

Research is showing that fluoride in drinking water does not make any difference to tooth decay and may cause a number of health issues, including damage to the brain, thyroid and bones.

In addition, today's vegetables are depleted in essential vitamins and minerals due to land being over farmed. Even organic vegetables are lower in nutrients in comparison to their counterparts from one hundred years ago.

Then there are processed foods, which are often loaded with sugar, or even worse, artificial sweeteners and trans fats. Many of these processed foods also contain manmade chemicals used as preservatives, colouring and flavourings. To complicate matters even further, the same brand of product can have different ingredients and additives when manufactured for a foreign market, due to differing food regulations. This is something to be aware of when travelling, as you may have no problem with a particular food product at home, but could be intolerant to it when purchased in a different country.

Doctors rarely tell you what is wrong with you is related to the food you are eating, or the environment in which you are living. Mainly because they are not taught this in medical school. Most diseases, including menopausal symptoms, are at least heavily influenced and often caused by an intolerance, or allergy to something you are ingesting.

Do you feel like you are doomed?

No, you are not doomed! This just means you need to be more aware and more selective than your grandparents used to be about what you eat and what you put on your body.

Over the next few pages I'm going to share with you what I've learnt about food and the toxic environment to which we unwittingly subject our bodies. I will also address what is a healthy diet and how to maintain health and an optimum weight. You can then make an informed decision on what is right for you and your family.

Intensive Farming

In the drive to produce readily available and cheap food, farming has become more and more intensive.

Hormones and Antibiotics

To increase yields, meat and milk products (depending where they are produced) contain growth hormones, steroids, antibiotics and various chemicals and pesticides. These are added to animal feed or injected into the animal. As they are not all eliminated they end up in our milk and meat and this then has an advers effect on your hormones.

Growth hormones have been banned in animals within the European Union, but are still used in the USA and elsewhere. These growth hormones are often synthetic versions of oestrogen, progesterone and testosterone.

As I've mentioned previously, your body is unable to process these synthetic hormones, so your body protects itself by laying down fat to store them. The same happens within animals, so as you ingest their fat you are getting a high dose of these chemicals. This can be a major contributor to why some people are unable to lose weight. These synthetic hormones also upset your natural hormone balance. This can result in menopausal symptoms and an increased risk of hormone related diseases, such as endometriosis and cancer of the breast and ovaries.

Antibiotics are fed to animals to keep them healthy in a crowded environment, but also to make them fat. Residues of these antibiotics remain in the meat and dairy products. Antibiotics are nondiscriminatory, killing off healthy as well as unhealthy bacteria in all areas of your body, but most importantly in the gut. This is why a course of antibiotics can often give you diarrhoea. The smaller amounts from food are unlikely to cause diarrohoea but they are having an adverse effect on your gut's bacteria, reducing diversity and the health of your gut. The bacteria in your gut influences how you absorb nutrients, burn off calories and stay lean. A good quality probiotic supplement can increase the quantity and diversity of your vital gut bacteria, boosting your health and natural immunity.

Scientists have discovered lean people have more good, anti-obesity bacteria in their guts than people who are overweight. A study of British children showed that those who had received many courses of antibiotics were more overweight than those who had received none or very few courses.

Antibiotics may be one of the reasons it is hard to lose those pounds or kilos. What is much scarier is their overuse, as this is increasing the danger of antibiotic resistant diseases such as MRSA (methicillin-resistant staphylococcus aureus).

Around 80% of antibiotics used in the USA are given to livestock. Since 1999 there has been a ban on the use of antibiotics to promote growth in livestock in Europe. Despite this ban, antibiotic use in UK agriculture only fell by 11% between 2004 and 2009.

You should therefore:

- Eat organic meat and dairy, which are hormone free and where antibiotics are only used when absolutely necessary to treat infection. Or know what your local farmer is using.

- Always have organic milk that is free from hormones and antibiotics.

- Avoid antibacterial soaps and hand wipes. Good old soap and water is just as effective and much better for your long-term health and wellbeing.

- Avoid taking antibiotics except if absolutely necessary and make sure you complete the whole course.

- Boost your immune system by eating healthily, spending time outdoors and taking a probiotic, plus vitamin D3 supplements during winter months, or if you spend a lot of time indoors.

Pesticides, Fungicides and Herbicides

Pesticides, fungicides and herbicides are sprayed on nearly all crops not grown organically, including fruit, vegetables, grains, nuts and seeds.

There are over 300 types of pesticide and many are extremely toxic. Despite so-called safe limits (often broken, especially on fruit) pesticides are doing untold damage to our bodies. They are not just on the outside of produce as some are systemic and thus are present throughout the whole vegetable or fruit.

An average person's annual intake of fruit and vegetables has had the equivalent of a gallon of pesticides sprayed onto it. Most pesticides are resistant to water, so washing fruit and vegetables before eating is ineffective.

Even though DDT has been banned since the 1970s, it still shows up regularly in fresh produce testing as soil is still contaminated by it. An expert committee who regularly tests foods for pesticide residues, has found 46% of current produce contains one or more pesticides, up from 25% in 2003.

Pesticides have been shown to be carcinogenic, but they also prevent your body from being able to defend itself against other carcinogens. Some of these chemicals imitate oestrogen and disrupt thyroid function, both of which can lead to weight gain and increase the risk of breast and ovarian cancer.

Pesticides have been linked with causing:

- Cancer
- Obesity (by slowing down metabolism)
- Parkinson's disease
- Diabetes
- Infertility
- Endometriosis
- Birth defects
- Autism
- Attention deficit disorder

- Respiratory disorders such as asthma

- Skin irritation

- Impaired immune system

- Kidney disease.

Pesticide Residues Found in Various Foods

Food type	% of samples containing residues	% of samples containing multiple residues
Citrus fruit	100	100
Pineapple	94	10.4
Apples	89	76
Grapes	88	70
Banana	57	38
Plums	23	5.6
Kiwi fruit	44	4.2
Tomatoes	81	52
Parsnips	77	67
Carrots	63	32

Sweet potatoes	57	6.4
Potatoes	44	8.3
Leeks	8	4.2
Onion	29	2
Spinach	47	22
Lettuce	59	27
Cereal grains	79-91	5.6

(Information taken from Pesticide Action Network UK)

Where possible, it is advisable to buy organic or locally produced seasonal crops. Local crops are likely to contain less chemicals, as they don't need to be preserved for long distance travel. Also crops that have been ripened by the sun have higher nutritional values than those picked unripened to allow for shipping and then ripened in store or after purchase.

If you live in the USA, avoid genetically modified crops such as wheat, corn, soy, canola and cottonseed used to produce oil often used in fast food restaurants. Your body doesn't know how to digest the changed proteins within the crops and they are also exposed to large amount of chemicals during growth and prior to harvesting. It is suspected that the large increase in the number of people suffering with coeliac disease and food intolerances is due to these practices.

High Fructose Corn Syrup

High fructose corn syrup is corn syrup which undergoes a process to increase its fructose content.

This substance is a major culprit in the obesity, diabetes, heart disease and cancer epidemic. It causes high levels of insulin production and blocks the hormone leptin, essential for appetite control. High fructose corn syrup fools your body into constantly thinking it is hungry.

It is found in a large proportion of processed foods including tomato ketchup, salad dressings, ice cream, yogurts, pasta sauces, frozen meals, beer and even in foods claimed to be healthy such as protein bars and natural sodas.

Just because a food is savoury it doesn't mean that it won't contain sugar.

It is estimated that an average person in the USA consumes 81g of high fructose corn syrup per day. A single standard glass of soda can contain 50g of high fructose corn syrup. In the UK according to Public Health England the average daily added sugar consumption of adults aged 19 to 64 is 58.8g. The recommendation is 25-30g daily.

Vegetable Oil

The government and medical profession have been advising us for years not to eat saturated fats, such as butter and coconut oil. We have been led to believe saturated fats raise blood cholesterol levels and increase the risk of heart disease. Instead, we were told to eat vegetable oils such as corn, canola/rapeseed, cottonseed, soybean and sunflower oil. These are classified as unsaturated, or polyunsaturated oils.

Vegetable oils have only been produced in the last 100 years. They are made by heating the grain and the use of toxic solvents and chemicals to extract the oil. These oils contain large amounts of Omega-6 fatty acids, which are harmful in excess as they cause inflammation - the route to nearly every disease. When used at high temperatures, many of these types of vegetable oil are also carcinogenic.

To make things even worse, these vegetable oils are often modified into trans fats, sometimes known as hydrogenated fats. They go through a process of hydrogenation to make them solid at room temperature, such as margarine.

Hydrogenated fats have been found to be highly toxic as they not only raise the level of bad (LDL) cholesterol, but also lower your good (HDL) cholesterol. They are now associated with increasing the risk of heart disease, diabetes, cancer and obesity.

Unfortunately, hydrogenated or trans fats are found in nearly all processed baked foods, including bread, biscuits, ready meals and fast food products.

As I write, the Food and Drug Administration (FDA) in the USA is taking action to reduce the amount of artificial trans fats in the food chain over the next three years. A ban is also been considered in the UK and Europe.

The belief that saturated fats cause heart disease is also being questioned. The French, Eskimos and people of northern India eat large amounts of saturated fats. The level of heart disease among these groups is lower than in countries where people eat little saturated fat.

Fats are essential to health. Your brain is made up of at least 60% fat. It has been suggested the increase in neurological diseases such as dementia, Parkinson's and Alzheimer's disease may partly be due to a low-fat diet and the wrong type of fat being consumed in the diet.

The best types of oil to consume are coconut, olive, nut, flaxseed and avocado which have been cold pressed and are preferably organic. Most of these oils are best used cold as heating them can make them become carcinogenic.

A good oil to use for cooking is organic, virgin coconut oil. It is also great on your skin and has some amazing properties. It is antibacterial, antiviral, anti-carcinogenic, anti-inflammatory and boosts the immune system.

Chemical Nutrition!

Additives

Grocery stores are full of processed foods and pretty much all of them contain additives to enhance colour, taste and act as preservatives. Some of these are natural but the majority are chemicals. When reading food labels, it feels like you need a degree in chemistry to understand them! You also have to attempt to translate a list of E numbers into the ingredients they really are.

To make an informed decision about what you are feeding yourself and your family, you need to become an avid label reader.

If you don't recognise an ingredient don't eat it.

Yes, it's a pain, if like me you have to dig out your reading glasses, but your health is your main asset so it's worth it!

Monosodium Glutamate (MSG)

MSG is a flavour enhancer found in many processed and fast foods as well as Chinese and Asian cuisine. It spices up bland food and makes it taste good as well as making you want more and more.

MSG can cause:

- Skin rashes

- Nausea

- Vomiting

- Headaches

- Asthma

- Depression

- Heart arrhythmias

- Obesity.

Artificial Sweeteners

There are a variety of artificial sweeteners on the market which have been introduced over the last forty to fifty years, thanks to the diet industry wanting a 'healthy' alternative to sugar. Many products, including soda and other soft drinks, switched to using sweeteners so they could advertise their products as 'sugar free.' Sweeteners include aspartame, saccharine, acesulfame K and sucralose. These products do not assist in you losing weight. Due to their toxic nature they could make you fat, or you might find it difficult to lose weight.

All these sweeteners have been found to be carcinogenic in their own right, or contain carcinogenic compounds. They can cause damage to the kidneys, intestinal upsets, skin rashes, tinnitus, joint pains and depression, to mention just a few of the potential side effects. Many of them are also classed as 'excitotoxins' and damage the brain and central nervous system, leading to impaired memory response and disturbance to neuroendocrine functions.

The manufacturers of goods using artificial sweeteners are aware of the bad press they are getting and are changing the names in the hope of disguising them. Aspartame is now labeled as 'Nutrasweet', 'Equal' or 'Aminosweet and is marketed as a natural sweetener. (It certainly is not natural!)'

There are now sweeteners on the market purported to be natural such as Stevia, but this can cause severe allergic reactions, digestive issues, dizziness, muscle pain and ovarian cancer.

For optimal health avoid all foods and drinks labelled as sugar free. They will do you more harm than the actual sugar variety, which should only be consumed in small amounts and not on a daily basis.

If you need a sweetener honey or maple syrup that has not been processed in any way are best.

Toxins

During the 1980s in the USA, the National Human Adipose Tissue Survey collected body fat samples from 1200 people. Their aim was to get a baseline of toxins in the body to monitor future clean up schemes. Frighteningly, every sample contained solvents, heavy metals, lead and mercury, plus toxic industrial pollutants.

Other studies have shown most of us have 400-800 chemicals stored in our fat cells, which can reside there for years. This can lead to chronic disease and hormone imbalance.

The body initially tries to flush out the toxins, but if toxins build up quicker than they can be eliminated, the body dilutes them and stores them in fat cells. As many toxins are fat soluble, more fat cells are produced as a way of protecting your vital organs from these chemicals.

Body fat around the midsection is often a sign of toxic build up and indicates that the liver is not functioning as efficiently as it should. It's not middle age spread!

Toxins can affect metabolism. They:

- Damage the mitochondria and reduce the cells' ability to burn sugar, which leads to disease and cancer.

- Reduce thyroid hormone levels, which is partly responsible for the basal metabolic rate (at rest) in fat and carbohydrate metabolism.

- Reduce the hormone leptin, which signals you are full.

- Act as an anti-nutrients. Stop nutrients being absorbed, or excrete nutrients before they've been absorbed.

A healthy liver is vital to help reduce the buildup of toxins in your body. Being overweight can damage your liver in the same way as consuming too much alcohol. As well as watching your weight, the milk thistle plant is excellent for supporting a healthy liver.

Petroleum

Petroleum not only keeps your car running, but is found in thousands of products including plastic, pesticides, clothing, medicines, solvents, soap, cosmetics and even perfume. It may have improved our quality of life in some ways, but it pollutes the environment and our body.

Petroleum is an endocrine disruptor and xenoestrogen, as it has an oestrogen-type effect on your body. It is fat soluble and non-biodegradable, so it can easily pass into the body and then sits there in your fat cells, wreaking havoc. It can cause infertility, feminisation of males, menopausal symptoms, endometriosis, cancer and suppression of the immune system.

Bisphenol-A (BPA)

The majority of us carry traces of BPA within our bodies.

It has been shown to cause hormonal changes in both men and women, as it increases oestrogen and therefore depletes progesterone and testosterone. In the early 20th century, one of its uses was to treat menopausal symptoms as it has a similar structure to oestrogen, before it was found to be carcinogenic and banned.

However, this did not stop BPA being used in the manufacturing of plastics and it is found in many products today including food containers. Even if you buy things that say they are BPA free, there are other Bisophenol like chemicals still in regular use.

Reducing Your Exposure to Chemicals and Toxins

It is impossible to avoid all chemicals and toxins as they are now such a major part of modern life, but you can reduce your exposure.

- Don't drink water or juice out of plastic bottles, especially if they have been exposed to heat or sunlight.

- Don't microwave plastic containers.

- Filter water for drinking and cooking.

- Eat organic.

- Use organic milk

- Avoid decaffeinated coffee and tea. Most are made by soaking the beans in ethyl acetate, or methylene chloride.

- Avoid fabric conditioners.

- Avoid scented products.

- Use natural aromatic oils instead.

- Use natural soaps, deodorants and cosmetics.

- If decorating or upgrading your home, make sure it is well ventilated and use natural paints and products.

- Avoid nail varnish and remover. (There are now a couple of brands that use natural oils).

- Become an expert at reading and understanding labels.

- Eat plenty of organic crucifer vegetables such as broccoli, cauliflower, cabbage and Brussels sprouts, as it has been suggested they neutralise excesses of oestrogen.

Food Intolerance and Allergies

Even foods classed as healthy can cause long-term health problems if they are not right for you. Everyone is unique and how you react to different foods is specific to you. Some negative effects are obvious, but others can be very subtle.

What you eat has an influence on many, if not all diseases, yet doctors rarely consider diet when making a diagnosis or deciding on treatment. This is because they receive very little training in nutrition.

Food allergies and intolerances are a growing concern the world over. According to Allergy UK there has been a 500% increase in hospital admissions for food allergies since 1990.

Over 150 million people in Europe have allergies and this is expected to rise to 50% of the European population by 2021. In the USA it is estimated that 15million people have food allergies.

The most common food allergies are:

- Peanuts
- Tree nuts - almonds, walnuts, cashews, pistachios, pecans
- Fish
- Shellfish
- Milk
- Eggs
- Wheat
- Gluten found in wheat, barley and rye.

Food allergies are easy to identify as your body has a huge abnormal immune reaction that can cause difficulty in breathing, swelling and hives. This often occurs within minutes of eating the food substance, makes you extremely ill and can even lead to death.

Food intolerance is harder to identify as the symptoms are subtler. Symptoms may not appear until hours after eating, or only if the substance is eaten in a large quantity, regularly, or in combination with another food.

Symptoms of food intolerances can be:

- Itching
- Skin rashes, eczema and dermatitis
- Headaches or migraine
- Aching joints
- Bloated stomach
- Loose stools or constipation
- Night sweats

- Hot flushes

- Irritable bowel

- Dark circles under the eyes.

It's likely you are intolerant to some foods if you are experiencing menopausal symptoms, or have any chronic condition such as asthma, eczema, or arthritis.

Identifying the foods I am intolerant to has helped me lose weight, stop hot flushes, reduce joint pain and have increased energy. On the odd occasion that I now get flushes, I can always relate them to stress or something I've eaten in the last few hours. White wine is unfortunately the biggest culprit.

The best way to test for food intolerances is to do an elimination diet for two weeks, in which you cut out the most common food culprits. In his book 'Diet Wise' Professor Keith Scott-Mumby suggests cutting out all dairy, eggs, grains, citrus fruits, tea, coffee, alcohol, or any manufactured food and essentially eat a 'paleo' diet of vegetables, fruit, fish and grass fed meat. After two weeks you gradually reintroduce foods one at a time and see if you have any adverse effects, such as an upset stomach, itching or headaches. Effects can be very subtle and not instantaneous, so closely monitor your body for 24 hours before trying another food. If you have any reaction leave the food out of your diet for at least a month before retesting.

It is possible to be tested for intolerances at a naturopathic clinic, though they are not as reliable as elimination and listening to or watching to see what your own body tells you. Blood tests performed at a doctor's surgery rarely show intolerances, only allergies.

One of the commonest intolerances is to modern wheat. The consumption of grains is very high in the average western diet - cereal for breakfast, a sandwich for lunch and pasta for supper is very common. Modern wheat is cultivated for high yields and contains thousands of different proteins, all of which can trigger sensitivity.

Small portions of the population are diagnosed with coeliac disease, an intolerance to the protein called gluten. Many people today are switching to gluten-free products, in the belief they are intolerant to gluten, but they are in fact intolerant to other proteins found in modern wheat that our bodies have not learnt to digest.

It has been suggested everybody may be sensitive to gluten or wheat proteins to some extent, without even knowing it.

Sensitivity can be responsible for headaches, tiredness, depression, anxiety, abdominal pain, black circles under the eyes, constipation or diarrhea. It increases the risk of a leaky gut, which in turn increases the inflammation process within your body.

Beware of gluten-free products, as they are often full of chemicals and sweeteners. As with all products you need to read the labels, even if it is a pain having to wear your reading glasses as you shop.

Glyphosate, a weed killer used heavily in the production of wheat, has been implicated in the rise in the number of people diagnosed with coeliac disease and it is likely to be affecting everyone else to some extent too.

To reduce menopausal symptoms and obtain optimal health, limit the amount of grain products you consume and switch to rye, oats and old flour types such as Spelt or Kamut.

Gut Microbes

A healthy digestive tract is essential for the digestion of food, but recent research shows that, "up to 90 percent of all known human illness can be traced back to an unhealthy gut" (David Perlmutter, MD; 2015).

You have around 10,000 types of microbes living within your body and you would not function without them. Most are found in your digestive tract and are responsible for breaking down the food you eat, so that it is available to your body. Bacteria are the most important microbes in maintaining your health and immune system. The health of your microbes can affect your brain functions, metabolism and even your libido and menopausal symptoms.

The types of food you eat and how stressed you are feeling determines the health of the microbes in your gut.

People with weight problems have been found to have different and less diverse gut flora to those of normal weight. Obesity can be classed as an inflammatory disease.

You are considered to be overweight with a body mass index (BMI), your weight relative to height, of 25 to 29.9. Obese refers to a BMI of 30 or higher.

Inflammation occurs due to a leaky gut. Your intestine is lined with a mucosal membrane, which allows broken down nutrients from your food to pass into your blood stream and prevents harmful particles from passing through. When the gut is leaking, it allows some of these harmful particles through. It is thought that food allergies, intolerances and the wrong balance of microbes due to poor diet, can cause the gut to leak.

To keep your gut healthy, eat foods such as garlic, Jerusalem artichoke and fermented food classed as prebiotic, along with food such as live yogurt that is probiotic. Prebiotics and probiotics can also be taken as a supplement, but ensure they are of high quality, as cheaper versions get destroyed by the acid in your stomach.

Healthy Eating

Whether you feel healthy, fit, energised and are able to maintain an ideal weight for your body type, is determined by what you eat. The best way to achieve this is through healthy eating of food that is right for your body's composition.

We are all unique, but this is rarely taken into consideration by the medical profession, scientists and media, when advising us what to eat. Trying to look like a supermodel who is naturally tall and lean, will be impossible to achieve if you have a body-type that naturally has broader shoulders and hips.

Some body types do well on a vegetarian, or raw food diet, whereas others require animal protein and food that has been heated. Even if a food is deemed healthy it might not be healthy for you. For example broccoli can cause skin problems and other issues in about six percent of the population.

However, for everyone a healthy diet consists of food that is fresh and unprocessed, preferably organic and contains no hydrogenated fats and little or no added sugar.

Following the latest diet fad that stipulates you must only eat cabbage, grapefruit, high protein, low fat or count the calories, rarely works in the long term. The result at best is yo-yoing between being the weight you want to be and being overweight.

In the UK about 11million people are on a diet at any one time, but over 80% of these diets fail.

Why Diets Don't Work!

- They don't take into consideration your own unique body's needs.

- Healthy eating needs to become a lifestyle choice, not just a quick fix.

- They make you feel deprived.

- You focus on what you can't eat.

- They depend on will power.

- Low calorie intake puts your body into starvation mode, so when you go on a crash diet or miss a meal, you end up holding on to fat, not losing it.

- They leave you feeling guilty when you don't follow the plan.

- They are often nutritionally imbalanced, so your body wants more food to get the correct nutrients.

- Special diet foods are often full of hidden ingredients and chemicals to maintain taste. Low fat foods are often very high in sugar and sugar free foods high in fat and toxic sweeteners.

Why Do You Overeat/Hold on to Weight?

- Automatic response to negative feelings.

- Comfort

- Childhood conditioning - having to eat everything on your plate.

- Guilt

- Habit

- Stress

- Buying the wrong kind of food with poor nutritional content.

- Not recognising hunger/full signs.

- Shift work

- Eating in front TV, computer.

- Low self-esteem

- Excess blood sugar

- Hormone imbalance

- Food intolerance

- Protection from abuse or because of past abuse.

- Medications

- Environmental toxins and chemicals in food.

Unfortunately, there is no magic wand for weight loss. Sometimes you don't need to lose weight, but you would look and feel better if some fat is converted into muscle.

It is important not to get fixated by what the scales tell you, as muscle weighs more than fat. Instead, go by how well your clothes fit, how much energy you have and how well you feel. Stop comparing yourself to others, it's what's right for you that counts!

Losing weight is not just about the food you put in your mouth, or even the exercise you do or don't do. Every aspect of your life and how you react to events can influence how easy or hard you find it to lose weight.

People who lose weight and then maintain it are not on a diet. They have learnt healthy habits around food and maintain a healthy lifestyle.

Start today and begin to establish a beneficial healthy relationship with food, with the sole purpose of nourishing your body. It's about small steps.

Start by recognising past emotions and habits around food.

Food Diary.

The first step towards healthy eating, losing weight and reducing hot flushes and night sweats is being aware of:

- *what you are eating when you reach for food*
- *what you are doing when you reach for food*
- *how you are feeling when you reach for food and drink on a daily, minute-by-minute basis.*

A good place to start is by keeping a food diary for a few days. It's easy to underestimate how much you actually eat. How you are feeling when you reach for food is probably something you are not even aware of.

By keeping a diary, you can see what habits you have around food, when you reach for food to get comfort and what you have eaten before experiencing a hot flush. A hot flush or night sweats may occur very quickly after eating, or it may be hours later, as you start to digest that food.

Keep a note of everything you eat and drink from the minute you wake up until you go to sleep. This is purely for your information, so be honest with yourself.

Just as important as what you are eating, is why? Eating between meals is often due to feeling sad, bored, feeling you deserve a treat, or just through sheer habit. The kids are in bed, your favourite TV programme is on, therefore it's time for a glass of wine and a packet of crisps. It's this type of eating that is often the culprit for most weight gain, rather than what you eat at mealtimes.

Keep a note of any possible food reactions, such as headaches, itchy skin, difficulty in sleeping, or exacerbation of menopausal symptoms.

Do this exercise on a couple of working days and over a weekend. Once you can see what it is you are eating, when and why, you can then begin to take small action steps in changing your eating habits.

Don't be overwhelmed, it's as simple as:

- *what*
- *when*
- *why*

It might take longer to be aware of what is triggering hot flushes and night sweats. Common culprits are alcohol, coffee and chocolate. Be aware that it might also be foods in combination - eating them on their own is fine, but put them together with something else and they are a problem.

Download A Food Diary
http://www.pamlob.com/food-diary/

Helpful Hints and Facts to Aid Weight Loss

You make over 200 decisions each day about food, based on emotions, habits, environment and the people you are with. Are you making the right decisions?

- Concentrate on natural foods. Eat organic as much as possible to reduce exposure to xenoestrogens.

- Try to eat carbohydrates such as bread and pasta before 3pm. Limit the amount of grain you eat by not eating it daily and only having it for one meal.

- Reduce sugar intake (sugar is highly addictive) as excess is converted to fat. Cancer feeds on sugar and it could be growing in your body without your knowledge.

- Eat a good breakfast.

- Eat four to six small meals per day, rather than one main meal late in the evening.

- Increase the amount of exercise in your life. It doesn't have to be going to the gym. Take the stairs, walk to work or park further away, walk faster, go for a short walk at break times.

- Get support to help with motivation and for accountability.

- Get plenty of sleep:
    - o Lack of sleep causes weight gain.
    - o Our bodies regenerate the most between 10pm and 2am.
    - o The longer you sleep in, the harder it is to lose weight.

- Drink plenty of water. If you feel thirsty you are already dehydrated.

- When you feel hungry, first drink a glass of water or a herbal tea (no milk) and then see how you feel. Your body finds it hard to differentiate between thirst and hunger.

- Plan meals in advance.

- Don't shop for food when you are hungry.

- Read food labels.

- Avoid processed food, takeaways and fizzy drinks.

- Don't see healthy eating as eliminating food. Find healthy food that you enjoy. There are some great cake recipes that are wheat, dairy and sugar free.

- Ask yourself, what is it you are really hungry for? It might be love, affection, praise etc. and not food. See food as fuel for your body, not something to get comfort from. Identify other activities that improve your mood, give you comfort and/or distract you.

- Make this change of lifestyle about **you**. Become interested in your relationship with food.

1) Eat mindfully (without distraction from TV) at least once a day, so that you pay attention to your body and hear the full messages.

- Eat till satisfied and then stop.

- Eat with enjoyment and pleasure.

- Avoid food advertisements as they hypnotise you into buying their products.

- Stop looking for substitutes - eat real food, instead of diet foods or those that are labelled 'reduced fat' or 'fat free,' as the fat is replaced by sugars or chemicals.

- Add turmeric, cinnamon, rosemary, oregano, garlic powder and paprika to dishes to boost your metabolic rate and benefit from their many healing properties.

Being overly thin can be as dangerous to your health as obesity. What is more important than your weight, is how healthy you feel and how active you are.

Vitamin and Mineral Supplements

If you are eating a nutritious, well-balanced diet you shouldn't need to take supplements, except vitamin D if you don't get enough strong sunlight in the winter months. However as already discussed, your diet isn't always able to provide all the vitamins and minerals you need for optimal health.

Before taking supplements, have your levels checked and discuss your needs with a health professional. If you are taking other medication always check with a pharmacist about adverse effects.

Vitamin B complex

This group of water-soluble vitamins may help you deal with the stress of menopausal symptoms, especially vitamin B6 and B12. They can help you deal with adrenal fatigue, brain fog and help with mood swings. Vitamin B6 may also help with weight loss.

Vitamin E

Vitamin E is an antioxidant that helps slow down damage to cells. A daily dose of natural vitamin E can help alleviate symptoms of hot flushes, vaginal dryness and can reduce the risk of heart attacks.

Vitamin C

Vitamin C is also an antioxidant that helps to boost the immune system, reduce hot flushes, vaginal dryness and help retain the elasticity in the urinary tract to prevent stress incontinence. It also helps to build up collagen to maintain skin elasticity and bone health.

Vitamin D - 'the sunshine vitamin'

Vitamin D is essential for good health, strong bones and immune system. Recent research shows that it is a key player in preventing and treating cancer and long-term health conditions.

Improved vitamin D levels can help your sexuality, increase testosterone and reduce stress and anxiety.

Unlike other vitamins, your body makes vitamin D from sunlight and only a very small proportion comes from food. Therefore, it is essential to get enough sunlight, or take a supplement.

Today a high proportion of the population in northern latitudes greater than 36° north, or southern latitudes less than 36° south, are deficient in vitamin D, many of them seriously. Two weeks holiday in the sun barely makes a dent in your levels.

Vitamin D deficiency occurs because:

- The sun is not strong enough during the winter months, along with wearing layers of clothes so very little skin is exposed.

- Sunscreen is worn all day during the summer months.

- People spend very little time outside.

- It is required daily and not enough can be obtained from food.

If you are fair-skinned, 10,000 international units of vitamin D are produced under your skin from being out in sunlight for just 30 minutes. The length of time your skin should be exposed to sunlight is about half the time it takes for your skin to turn pink. The more skin you expose, the more vitamin D you produce.

The darker your skin, the longer exposure time you need to produce the same levels of vitamin D as someone who is fair. Therefore, people who are dark-skinned and live in northern or southern latitudes, are more likely to require vitamin D supplements for a longer period.

Research on the effectiveness of sunscreen in the prevention of skin cancer is producing mixed results. Most sunscreens are also full of chemicals. Factor 50 sunscreen, or total sunblock, is the most damaging due to the type of chemicals used to block the sunlight.

The safest way to protect yourself from sun damage is to cover up your skin with protective clothing, don't forget a brimmed hat, or stay in the shade between the hours of 11am and 3pm. (This may be longer if you are very fair, or are close to the equator).

If you are unable to get enough Vitamin D daily from sunlight, then supplementation is often essential even during the summer months. You can get your vitamin D levels checked by your doctor to see how much supplementation you require. Have your levels checked at least once a year to ensure they are within healthy and safe limits.

The best type of Vitamin D to take is Vitamin D3 as this is the same vitamin produced naturally by your body. If you get vitamin D prescribed by your doctor, it is likely to be Vitamin D2, so ask for D3, or buy your own. The Vitamin D Council recommends taking 5,000IU and no more than 10,000IU daily. This should be split into two doses, taken morning and evening with your meals.

As with all supplements, if you are taking medication, check with a pharmacist that it is safe to take vitamin D.

To help with the absorption of vitamin D, you should also take vitamin K2 (MK7). Take 100mcg to 200 mcg per day, in order to assist in the process of sending calcium back into the bones.

Magnesium

Magnesium is a mineral found in large quantities in the body where it is involved in over 300 chemical reactions. Deficiency can cause muscle cramps, menstrual cramps, poor sleep, anxiety, headaches, osteoporosis, depression, chronic pain and chronic fatigue syndrome.

Many people are depleted in this mineral due to drinking carbonated drinks, eating foods high in sugar, caffeinated drinks, stress and taking calcium supplements without added magnesium.

Foods high in magnesium include green leafy vegetables, sea vegetables, beans, nuts, fish and whole grains. However, it is hard to achieve adequate levels from diet alone.

The best form of magnesium to take as an oral supplement is magnesium citrate, glycinate taurate, or aspartate, at a dose of 400 to 1,000mg per day. Avoid magnesium carbonate, sulfate, gluconate or oxide, as they are poorly absorbed. As magnesium is a great relaxant, a good time to take it is before bed, however on a higher dose it is best taken twice daily. Supplementation can cause diarrhoea.

Research is suggesting that taking it transdermally (sprayed onto your skin) as magnesium oil has better absorption. Oil can be bought ready-made, or a cheaper alternative is magnesium chloride flakes dissolved in distilled water in a spray bottle. Epsom salt baths are also an excellent way to increase your intake and it's a great way to relax as well.

Redox Cell Signaling Supplement

For optimal health we need healthy cells that are working efficiently and correctly. One of the fastest growing areas of science in the world is in Redox signaling and scientists are saying it's as big a discovery as DNA. James Watson, the Nobel Prize Winner for his work on DNA, suggests many major diseases are caused by the lack of Redox signaling molecules.

Redox signaling molecules are produced by the mitochondria and are essential to cellular health and cell communication internally and between each cell. A way to understand the process is to see the mitochondria as a fireplace. When everything is working optimally energy and Redox signaling molecules are produced. If it's not burning correctly the smoke enters the room, or cell in this instance, and this causes oxidation. Redox molecules then signal to the fire brigade (the antioxidants, immune system and hormones) that assistance is needed to put out the fire and return to health. If the fire brigade is unable to repair the cell it signals for atoposis (cell death) to occur and a good quality new replacement to be made.

However, the body's supply of Redox signalling molecules decreases with age and through disease. Lack of signaling means the fire brigade does not receive the call for help and instead of the cell being repaired or atoposis occurring, when the cell divides the damage is replicated and signs of aging and disease occur.

To maintain the health of your cells and the production of Redox signalling molecules your body requires a healthy environment internally and externally, including a good diet, the right exercise and limited stress.

The good news is it's also now possible to take a supplement to replace and stimulate your Redox signalling molecules. Research has shown that taking a supplement can switch on the gene pathways that:

- Improve your immune system
- Modulate hormone balance
- Improve gut health and digestive enzyme production
- Help maintain cardiovascular health
- Help maintain a healthy inflammatory response.

If you want to know more, please visit my website http://pamlob.teamasea.com/
or contact me for more information.

Personalise What You Eat and Your Life

Your life and your future are not predetermined.

Every one of us is unique, even identical twins with the same genetic profile. This means there is no one size fits all answer to losing weight, exercising or curing disease. Yet this is the approach of the medical, health, fitness and diet industry.

This is why obesity and chronic disease are on the rise despite all the scientific breakthroughs of the last few years. If a diet or treatment for a chronic disease has worked for you it's often more through luck than judgement.

When the human genome was first sequenced, it was thought it would put an end to disease as who you are, the way your body looks and functions and how your mind works is all influenced by your genes. Your genes are unique to you except if you are an identical twin. However, it has turned out to not be that simple as having a gene for a specific disease does not mean you will get that disease.

Our genes are just a blueprint. They are like the script to a play. It is the environment, our epigenetics both inside and outside our bodies, that determines how a gene is expressed. With a script for a play how it turns out depends on the director and the actor's interpretation of the script. If you go and see the same play night after night, there will always be subtle differences. This environmental switching of gene pathways on and off is why identical twins can end up looking very different and why only one develops a disease. This is the epigenetics effect.

Everything that goes on outside and inside of your body influences your health. This includes your lifestyle, the type of work you do, where you live and what you put into your body in the form of nutrients and chemicals. Even the time of day you eat, exercise and sleep has an effect. To a large degree you have the choice of what you subject your body to, so this means just because your mother had menopausal symptoms and your father has heart disease, it doesn't mean you will, even if you have that genetic marker. By just changing your environment to one which is right for you, can make big changes to your health and wellbeing.

I thought I was living a healthy life, eating nutritious food, avoiding food I was intolerant to, reducing my chemical exposure as much as possible, doing moderate exercise and keeping stress to the minimum. I had come to terms with the fact I was never going to have endless energy or lose any significant weight.

However, when I started following a personalised health plan with foods specific to my body's present needs, my energy very quickly soared to levels I had last experienced in my twenties. A great bonus was I dropped four dress sizes in six months and now look and feel better, well beyond my wildest dreams!

None of the changes I made were drastic. In fact I started eating again foods I had omitted from my diet, believing I was intolerant to them. Finding out the right physical environment for me is probably one of the things that has made the biggest difference to my energy. My body, it turns out, likes it hot and dry, so I live in England!

I've found that when I go to the right climate, like Denver in the summer, I can hike up mountains easier than I can my local Peak District hills. To cope with the English climate I've recently moved into a new house that is easy to keep warm and I'm decorating in warm colours. My body is very grateful!

Knowing the right environment, including the right foods and exercise for your unique needs is essential. Equally, who to socialise with and the most effective way to use your mind and talents. Even what time of day to eat, exercise and rest, the best climate to live or holiday in, can support you not just in ridding your body of menopausal symptoms, but also in improving your overall health and wellbeing.

In this chapter and within this book, I've already given you some ideas to start making changes in your life.

If you want to find out what your unique needs are and have a personal health plan designed just for you, without the need for expensive and invasive blood tests, please visit:

http://www.pamlob.com/personalised-health.

CHAPTER 4

Why Your Beliefs Are Sabotaging You

"Your beliefs become your thoughts. Your thoughts become your words. Your words become your actions. Your actions become your habits. Your habits become your values. Your values become your destiny."

Mahatma Gandi

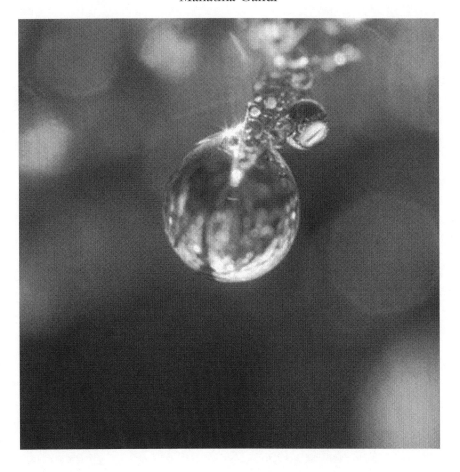

WHY YOUR BELIEFS ARE SABOTAGING YOU

WATCH Why Your Beliefs are Sabotaging You
http://www.pamlob.com/why-your-beliefs/

Your mind is incredibly powerful and used in the right way, alongside the right diet and lifestyle, it can help cure cancer and other diseases. Used in the wrong way, it can attract negative experiences into your life and lead to your demise. Over the years I've seen and heard of many people who are still alive after a terminal diagnosis and their lives transformed by a near death expereince. One of the best books I have read on this subject is Anita Majoorani's book 'Dying to be Me'. I also know of others who had been given a clean bill of health, but died anyway as they had given up the will to live.

If you believe that as you transition through midlife you will have menopausal symptoms, you are guaranteed to experience some menopausal symptoms!

The more you resist, or deny your menopausal symptoms, or anything else for that matter, the worse they are likely to get. As the energy of resisting something causes it to persist and even get stronger. Therefore, if you believe that menopause is a natural transition, you are less likely to have any symptoms, especially if other areas of your life, such as your attitudes to stress and eating a healthy diet, are also in alignment.

Many women dread turning forty, seeing it as the point of leaving their childbearing years behind them. Many see forty as the start of the slippery, downhill slope of worsening health, energy and cognitive function, until the day they turn up their toes and leave this life forever. Others see it as, 'life begins at forty.'

Take a moment and look at your beliefs about menopause and diseases that run in your family.

What You Believe Affects What You Attract Into Your Life

There is a saying 'you are as old as you feel.'

There is some truth in this, as your biological age has nothing to do with the chronological age found on your birth certificate. A young girl of eighteen with anorexia can have bones riddled with osteoporosis, to the level that you'd expect to see in somebody in their eighties. Whereas an eighty-year-old who is fit and healthy can have the body of someone half their age, or younger.

What you believe your body will be like at a certain age is more important than your genes on determining your ageing process. Your body is renewed every seven years and some cells are renewed daily. Therefore, if you take care of your health and wellbeing, it is possible to lower your biological age and reverse any damage.

You may believe because heart disease, osteoporosis, or cancer runs in your family, you therefore stand a very high chance of suffering with one or more of these diseases.

Some diseases are hereditary, or familial and if they exist in your family, there is a risk that you will have inherited the genes that predispose you to these diseases. But having the gene doesn't determine you will get the disease. To get the disease, that gene or several genes need to be switched on. It is your epigenetics, the things outside your genes such as the environment, your diet and beliefs, that determine which way the switch will fall. It's possible to switch genes on and off, by changing your lifestyle and thoughts.

If you believe that something will happen, especially if it is emotionally charged, it is more likely it will. This is the Law of Attraction.

Who you think you are is how you will show up in life!

Midlife Brain Changes

During menopause many women complain of brain fog and irritability. This may be due to the fact the brain chemistry of how you think and process information is changing. Brain chemistry changes at puberty and menopause, hence the unstable mood swings at these times.

As they move on from menopausal symptoms and the fog clears, women report they have stronger feelings about unfairness and injustice, greater creativity and renewed passion for making a mark in the world. If brain fog continues it is likely due to a food intolerance, particularly wheat.

Menopause is a great time to let go of limiting beliefs, step out of your comfort zone into the 'River of Life' and follow your dreams.

You Are NOT Your Beliefs

You are an energetic being made up of body, emotions, mind and spirit, known as your higher self, or your intuition. Your conscious mind is very powerful, yet it is only a very small part of who you are.

Our education system and western culture has made many people believe that our conscious mind is the dominant organ of our being. The result is you are only using a small percentage of what is available to you. Just imagine how amazing life could be if you increased this percentage. To do this, you need to connect to the whole of you, especially your heart, (more on this later in this chapter) not just your headspace.

Body and emotional awareness is essential to transform the mind.

Watch a baby or young child and you instantly see how well they are connected to their bodies and emotions. They learn through movement and play, they allow emotions to move quickly through them, one minute playing happily, the next throwing a temper tantrum to express anger and the next laughing.

As you grow through childhood your parents and teachers tell you it is wrong to cry whenever you are upset, or throw a temper tantrum when you are angry. Then you go to school and have to sit for hours behind a desk, being told you must sit still and concentrate, when what you really want to do is run around and explore. In order to meet these requirements, you disconnect from your body, emotions and energy. You develop defensive blocks to stop you feeling bad and keep you feeling safe.

These blocks have resulted in the majority of people living life from their headspace. They feel guilty about the past, worrying about tomorrow, or what to cook for tea, rather than enjoying the present moment. It is this disconnect from the present and a lack of awareness of the whole of you which keeps you stuck, living in a 'pond' rather than experiencing the delights of living in the 'River of Life.'

This disconnect from the whole of you is exacerbated by bombardment from an endless 'To Do' list, emails that demand immediate attention and the constant drip feed of social media, along with others constantly demanding your attention. When you are overwhelmed and pulled in lots of different directions, your mind is cluttered and you will never have the calmness and relaxation you crave. Instead you are likely to:

- Feel anxious.

- Worry constantly over minor things.

- Have low energy.

- Have poor focus.

- Take longer to do things.

- Are not present in the 'now.'

- Find it hard to sleep, or wake in the middle of the night and are unable to get back to sleep.

Your Subconscious Mind

Your conscious mind is like the 10% of an iceberg you can see above sea level. Your subconscious mind is the 90% you cannot see.

The conscious mind is controllable, it helps you generate thoughts, ideas and decisions. It is the translator of the messages from your subconscious, heart, gut, nervous system and intuition.

Your subconscious mind is like a filing cabinet, or computer hard disc. It controls 96-98% of your perception and behaviour. It is the storage of all your experiences, images, habits and beliefs. The subconscious mind operates everything you do automatically, from being able to walk, to driving a car, or how you respond to a situation.

The subconscious mind works only in the 'now' and cannot tell the difference between real and imagined, which is why visualisation can be so powerful. It also cannot tell the difference between the truth and a lie, so be careful what you tell yourself.

To understand how the conscious and subconscious mind interact, it is helpful to know a little about how your brain works in different mental states. The different brainwave frequencies are:

Alpha

Relaxation, or flow states. A slow alpha state is the twilight zone between being awake and being asleep. Whereas a higher alpha is when you are totally involved with what you are doing. This state is associated with joy, happiness, peace and positivity. It is the primary state in meditation.

Beta

Normal waking consciousness. You probably spend most of your day in beta mode, as it is associated with concentration and cognition. If your beta waves are operating more rapidly, you can feel anxiety and disharmony.

Delta

Deep sleep. Experts in meditation can remain alert in this state.

Theta

Creativity and dreaming. Theta is the state of hypnosis and visualisation, the channel to your subconscious mind. All hypnosis is self-hypnosis, a hypnotherapist is merely a guide. If your subconscious mind doesn't want you to do something, you will come out of hypnosis, or it won't work.

When you are in a theta state, you can be very creative, able to problem solve easily and soak up information. Theta also gives you access to awareness, showing you a new perspective of yourself or a situation.

Unfortunately, most people only experience Theta waves when they are asleep as they don't give themselves the time and space to relax.

You are not born with beliefs and habits. They develop as you grow and are socialised into society. During the first seven years of your life, you operate primarily in a theta state, absorbing automatically all that goes on around you into your subconscious mind. This is a great way to learn, but the downside is you are taking in the beliefs and behaviours of everyone around you, whether they are helpful to you or not. After seven years of age, you start operating more from the conscious mind. You are able to choose what it is you want to do, have and feel, if you are operating from a place of awareness.

A major issue on changing your beliefs, is you only operate from your conscious mind less than 5% of the time. As soon as your conscious mind thinks about the past, or the future - when you go into story mode, your conscious mind is unable to recognise what it is you want or need right now. It instead defaults to your subconscious mind, where most of the programming has come from someone else, or a much younger, more simplified you.

Become aware of your mind going into story, or judgement mode, and consciously listen to the words and sentences you are using to tell yourself what to do next.

Many of them are laughable and some are just sad, negative and even dangerous! Become aware whether the words are from your adult or your child persona.

Psychologists suggest 70% of our subconscious programming disempowers us.

When you operate from the subconscious, those around you may be aware of your disempowering behaviour, but you are blind to it. This can cause a disconnection, or a feeling of uneasiness between yourself and another.

To prevent defaulting to the subconscious, you need to remain mindful and aware of what's going on around you and what you want in each given moment. A want is not a new Ferrari or a pair of Jimmy Choos.

The next new shiny object, the material things don't make you happy for more than a few minutes. Happiness comes from within, it's what your heart tells you that you want right now. It could be as simple as a cup of tea, to go to the bathroom, or to take a break. Why your heart? I'll explain in a moment.

However, there will still be plenty of times you default into the subconscious, therefore it is important to reprogram the subconscious mind of negative thinking patterns, beliefs and habits that don't serve you.

Many people try to achieve this by talking to themselves, telling themselves not to act or talk this way. But the subconscious mind does not recognise the words 'you' or 'don't'. It's just a program that replays automatically when called for. The conscious mind can learn from reading a self-help book like this one, but the subconscious mind does not learn that easily, as it is there to protect you.

To recognise limiting beliefs:

Look down at yourself as if from a helicopter flying above your head, or think about how you would respond to a friend who was having a similar issue. This is a great way of overcoming your limiting belief and recognising your own value.

Ask yourself questions such as:

"Is this true for me and my life right now?"

To reprogramme the subconscious, you can use:

- Hypnosis: listen to recordings that assist the brain to go into a theta state.

- Habituation: constantly practicing and repeating a behaviour, just like you did when you were learning to drive, or learning to read.

- Visualisation: works like hypnosis but you are, see and more importantly feel an experience you want to achieve. The visualisation needs to be as if the experience is happening in the present moment. The more feeling and emotion you bring into play, the more effective it will be. The subconscious mind is unable to tell the difference between an actual experience and an imagined experience, so visualisation can be even more powerful than hypnosis scripts as the words, visions and emotions they evoke are yours.

- Meditation: regularly practicing meditation helps you access more easily and readily your alpha and theta states.

- Positive affirmations: repeat positive present state statements such as, "I am successful, I am beautiful, I have peace in my life."

Positive affirmations can be tricky and may unconsciously elicit the opposite, as it may be too far to stretch to believe the affirmation.

For example:

"My back is healing," will work, as it is a progressive process.

Whereas: "My back is healed," may cause your mind to say, "no that is not true."

The Power of Words

Every thought you have is tied to a string of words. These words are so incredibly powerful! They can influence your genes - such as those that regulate your stress response. When you have a negative thought, or are coming from a stressed position, the fear part of your brain becomes active and causes the frontal lobe to become less active. This effects how you speak, and you can sound more irritable and tension appears in your facial muscles. This causes a defensive reaction in your listener and has negative effects on your relationships.

Relationships are built from good communication, but what is frequently overlooked is how you communicate with yourself. You have an internal voice that chatters away voicing your thoughts. Telling you what to do, what not to do, that you are not good enough etc. These subconscious negative thoughts can leak out in your body language and lead to a listener thinking you are inauthentic.

How often do you really listen to what your internal voice is saying?

This voice can often be negative, mean, belittling and self-deprecating. The meanings that you have assigned to words are often not true, though you believe they are. These meanings then lead to negative outcomes and reinforce negative beliefs, such as, "I am a failure, I'll never succeed, I'm not worthy," etc. They become a self-fulfilling prophecy.

As you listen, ask yourself whether you would talk to others in this manner?

My guess is your answer would be "No way." So why are you talking to yourself in such a way that is destroying your self-esteem and confidence?

You do have control over the words spoken by your mind, it just feels at times as if you don't! You have the choice to believe or dismiss what it is telling you. The more you dismiss it, by taking your awareness to your body and how you are feeling right NOW, the easier it becomes to change the thoughts to a positive, or put things into perspective.

The voice in your head should be a translator of how you are feeling in the now, both good and bad, positive and negative, along with what your heart and intuition is telling you. The voice should not be a storyteller that keeps you stuck in the past, or worrying about the future.

Most people see the meaning of a word as a picture, a feeling, or an action. When you say or hear the word 'table' you see something with legs and a flat surface. In western culture you recognise 'yes' as a nod and 'no' as a shake of the head. The mind doesn't recognise words such as 'don't' or 'can't.' In order not to see or feel something, your mind first has to feel or see it before trying to erase it. Therefore, what happens is you are reinforcing what it is you don't want.

For example...

If I said to you, "Don't look at the elephant in the corner," what do you instantly see? An elephant in a corner! This means if you are in pain, every time you think, "Ouch I'm in pain," you are reinforcing it and eventually it becomes chronic as 'neurons that fire together, wire together.' Therefore, you can be experiencing pain even though there is no longer anything physically wrong.

It is possible to reverse chronic pain and even cure cancer by telling yourself you are healing and using positive language, rather than using negative words like pain, or cancer.

I used to have chronic lower back pain, from an injury that occurred when I was nursing. I had back pain for over 20 years, despite regularly seeing a physiotherapist, osteopath and chiropractor. Physically, there was no longer anything really wrong with my back, but I had focused for so long on pain the neurons in my brain had become wired for pain at that point in my back.

I then discovered the power of my mind and realised my back was literally holding me back! Once I had the awareness, whenever I felt pain in my back instead of saying 'my back is painful,' I switched it to 'my back is healing.' It took about three months but I no longer have chronic pain. My back is no longer preventing me from doing things I want to do. Back pain will still occur when I am stepping up to something new, my fear comes through physically. I just say "thank you for wanting to keep me safe" and then I take action towards my goal. Life had become so much more joyful and exhilarating now I no longer play small and safe.

I know now that the 'Law of Attraction' simply gives you what you are thinking of the most.

The Law of Attraction

You might not want to believe it, but you are responsible for what happens in your life. Blaming others is a defence block. You are constantly sending out waves of energy into the universe and this energy can act as a magnet. If you are sending out negative energy, then that is what will come back to you.

However, the 'Law of Attraction' does not mean you only have to think positively about a million pounds and it will miraculously turn up in your bank account. If only it was that easy! It requires awareness, focus and action.

Your past thoughts, habits and beliefs are responsible for how you react to what is happening in the now. Everything you focus on now will determine your future, so by changing your focus in the now, you can change a future outcome.

Negative thoughts are always going to pop up, as they are there to keep you safe. It is you who chooses whether you want to listen to them and be ruled by them, or take another route.

To take another route, you need to first be aware of your thought and you need to pay attention to your body, emotions, energy and intuition.

Change comes from commitment, not just interest. If you are just interested, excuses and stories will keep you stuck where you are. If you commit, you will take the action towards change. The action steps don't have to be huge, in fact small steps are often more successful.

As you read this book are you just interested in what I write? You might learn some new facts, but nothing will change until you commit to taking action to transform your health, wellbeing and relationships.

The Power of Your Heart

Many people only think of the heart in two ways:

- A pump that pumps the blood around your body to keep you alive.

- A symbol of love.

But your heart is so much more. And **yes, it can think**!

Research by The Heart Math organisation has shown your heart has its own energy field that is about sixty times stronger than the energy field of the brain. It has its own nervous system and more messages are passed from the heart to the brain than vice versa, but our mind and ego overrides a lot of this information.

Your heart is your core. It's the first organ that develops as a foetus and is the centre of your feelings, electromagnetic energy and intuition, the communications centre of your soul and yes, love.

Positive feelings can create a harmonious heart rhythm that spreads throughout your body, improving health and wellbeing by balancing your nervous system. This will even transmit to those around you, helping them feel more balanced too.

By learning to listen less to your mind and reducing the power of your ego, you are able to connect with and hear your heart centre and intuitive voice.

Research is showing that by intentionally connecting to your heart centre and feeling love, compassion, care and a positive view of emotions, you can improve your health, relationships and wellbeing. The greatest gift you can give to yourself and the world is to become emotionally healthy, connected to self and able to connect with others.

Heart Intelligence is ...

"The art of feeling more joy in your life, through the process of accepting who you are, as you are, without making yourself wrong."

Christian Pankhurst -Heart IQ™

It's a practice for learning to:

- Open your heart by being aware of who you are in the world and by receiving from others.

- Listen to your heart by pausing and getting still. You can then connect with and feel your body, emotions, energy and mind. You are able to listen to your intuition and discern what it is you want right now. This can be as simple as a hug, wanting a cup of tea, or to go to the bathroom. It can also help you to be aware of your deepest longing.

- Follow your heart by taking action towards what it is you want and to develop the attitudes, such as trust, courage and willingness, that will support you in fulfilling your dreams.

When these are in place, you are able to communicate from your heart and build authentic, loving relationships.

The focus of heart intelligence is on joy and living an authentic life, true to who you really are. It's about loving yourself, the amazing, wonderful, perfect **YOU** and comes from the premise that...

'There is nothing wrong with you."

I can hear you shout as you read this statement, "Oh yes there is...."

"I am hot and sweaty, struggling with the menopause."

"I don't sleep well."

"My husband left me for his secretary."

"I'm overweight."

"I'm in constant pain."

All these statements and any like them are related to something going on in your life right now, or effecting only a small part of you. They are not who you are at your core. They don't define **who you truly are**.

It is easy to associate yourself with what's going on in your life, especially when it is something negative. It can feel like it is taking over your whole being.

The core of all of us is intrinsically good. Life events can wound us, and some of these events will permanently change us. However, your intrinsic goodness always remains intact and accessible when you receive the right support.

So keep reminding yourself throughout the day as negative statements arise:

"There is nothing wrong with ME."

We are taught from a young age it is wrong to feel certain emotions. Emotions like anger or sadness are common emotions thought of as negative emotions. When you attach shame, guilt or judgment to an emotion, it can feel negative. It is not the emotion itself that is negative.

Even when you deny or repress what you are truly feeling, the body still feels it. These denied feelings become part of your cellular memory and cause this memory bank to become overloaded. Your cells become like a pressure cooker that is unable to vent. It will eventually explode, sometimes as an explosion of rage, or hatred, or as an illness including depression, cancer and heart disease.

Our emotions are like a rainbow. Without all the colours there is no rainbow and to be whole and healthy, we need all our emotions. By just sitting with them, or expressing them from a place of safety as they arise, the emotion will pass quickly through you and won't cause violent outbursts, or long-term damage to your body. If you don't feel one side of the spectrum of an emotion, it is hard to feel the other. Without anger, you have no passion. Without sadness, it's hard to feel happiness.

Don't confuse emotions and feelings. Emotions come from within the body, they just pop up in response to a situation, like being scared in a haunted house when something jumps out at you.

Feelings, on the other hand, are the story your mind tells about the emotion or experience. So when you are sitting at home and all is safe, but you suddenly feel scared, that comes from your mind. It's hard to control emotions other than denying them, but they still have a habit of erupting like a pressure cooker letting off steam. You can easily change how you feel by just switching your attention to something else.

By learning how to expand your emotional range and express your emotions safely, it is possible to find positivity and joy - even in the emotions you are inclined to think of as negative. Your life can become amazing!

Learning 'heart intelligence' has transformed my life tremendously. I feel lighter, freer, connected with my body, emotions and energy. From there I am able to listen to my intuition and recognise what it is I really want. It has given me the courage to step out of my comfort zone in so many ways there is not space to mention them here.

But I now travel without fear, I love meeting new people and doing new things. By letting go of my limiting beliefs - not being good enough, clever enough, worthy enough - I have had the courage to set up my own business and to write this book.

I would love to teach you how to connect with your heart and have loads of joy in your life every day, so get in touch www.pamlob.com/contact and start transforming your life today.

Shadows and Defensive Blocks

As a young child you are unable to discern between feeling bad and being bad, as the sense of self has not yet developed. Your under-developed mind believes if it is feeling bad, there must be something wrong with who you are and core unworthiness is born.

This leads to you suppressing aspects of yourself you believe at this young age are bad, or not ok, and therefore something is wrong with you. To prevent others from seeing something is wrong with you, these beliefs become your shadows. You are not consciously aware of them, but they are an integral part of who you are.

What stops you from recognising and releasing these shadows is fear. Fear of who you really are and what you would find if you dared to take a look. This fear is so entrenched you will do anything to keep it hidden. Therefore you develop a persona, a mask to hide your true authentic self.

A good analogy is your body is a house. Within this house, there are a series of boxes, or even rooms that are locked. Possibly hundreds of rooms are locked, bolted and guarded to stop anyone else seeing inside them, as you are ashamed of what they contain.

You believe they contain things not acceptable to your family and friends. Things like:

- I'm not OK

- I'm not worthy

- I'm stupid

- I'm not loveable.

By suppressing these so called dark shadows, you also struggle in connecting with their opposing light shadows:

- I am beautiful

- I am successful

- I am clever

- I am worthy

- I am loveable.

In the belief you can stop others seeing your shadows and finding out how bad you are, you build defensive blocks to keep you safe and to distance yourself from unpleasant thoughts, behaviours and feelings. When these defences kick in, an exaggerated expression of the shadow sneaks out at the most inopportune moment, such as when you are stressed, or triggered by someone else's behaviour.

We all have loads of shadows and blocks, but some are stronger than others.

The attributes of a defensive block are useful, but when used in defence they are taken to an extreme. Therefore you don't want to get rid of them, just turn the energy of them up or down, as you would the volume on a radio.

But you do want to be rid of the judgements that keep them in place.

A powerful one for me is 'independence.' A great attribute to have, as it helps me stand on my own two feet and get on in the world without constantly asking for help. It makes me good at problem solving, but in the extreme it prevents me from asking for help. I will battle on, on my own, making myself ill. It also results in me isolating myself and rejecting others.

When my husband was ill with leukaemia, this was particularly strong, as I was constantly in a place of stress. I can now see that this particular time of my life would have been easier and pleasanter if I had accepted or asked for more help. Not only did I put more stress on myself, I also hurt and pushed away friends and family who wanted to assist and be a bigger part of our lives.

Your shadows and defensive blocks hold the key to your authentic self and hold some great gifts, once you've identified and embraced them. Therefore you don't want to hide them, but acknowledge and welcome them.

When you open the door to the long-locked room, what you find is something beautiful, but dusty, which with the windows open and a good cleaning can become a prized part of your home.

If they are hidden how do you find them?

1. Ask a friend or loved one, they are not as well hidden as you think they are.
2. Recognise the behaviours in others which trigger and annoy you, or what you admire. This comes from the mirror principle - you can only see in others what you have within yourself.
3. Childhood memories which are particularly vivid often hold important clues.

For me, friends highlighted independence and my fear of being needy to me after my husband's death. I was then able to recognise it probably started on the day my sister was born. My mother had a home birth, so when she went into labour I was sent next door to stay with a neighbour who I didn't know well.

Up until that point I had never been left with anyone other than close family and I had no idea why I'd been sent next door. I believed in that moment I'd been naughty and was therefore unlovable, stupid, unworthy and definitely not OK. The proof was I'd been abandoned!

From all the knowledge of a four-year-old, I worked out the only way not to feel this pain of abandonment and hide all these things that were obviously wrong with me, was to prove to myself and my parents I didn't need them. I could look after myself.

Once a defensive block is in place, you are constantly looking for proof that the reason you set it up is true. My independence was strengthened by going home and finding out I was no longer the centre of attention. It was reinforced again when I had to start school and my sister was able to stay at home with Mum.

There are likely to be many other life events that made me feel abandoned, or my achievements were not recognised, which reinforced this need to be independent and added to my stash of shadows.

When a defence mechanism is in play, it keeps you stuck and unable to be connected to your internal guidance system that tells you what it is you want in order to take action and move forward. It's like being stuck in a tunnel and unable to connect to the satellite that tells your car GPS system whether you need to go straight on, turn left or turn right to get to your destination.

So how do you get out of your 'tunnel' and get back on your way?

Christian Pankhurst founder of Heart IQ™ suggests you need:

- Safety
- Trust
- Understanding
- Awareness
- Relaxation
- Tenderness.

Once you've identified a defence block, you don't need to remove it from your life as it can have many positive attributes. Instead, play with turning the volume dial up or down.

- With independence issues, you should turn the volume down and be less controlling by asking for help more often.
- If you are needy, you should turn it up and practice being more independent.

Once you've identified a shadow, spend time examining how it has affected your life and what the gifts are within it. Don't work on too many at a time, one dark and one light is enough. It's a fun exercise to do with friends as you can help each other see how it has been running you and identify what the gifts are. These gifts are not always obvious and sometimes you need to really think outside the box.

The Mirror Principle

The world is your mirror. If you see something in another you like or dislike, it must be within you even if you are not aware of it, or would rather deny it.

We are energetic beings connected to all the other energy within the universe. The idea we are separate is just an optical illusion. Therefore, how you treat others determines how they treat you and how you treat yourself will also determine how others react to you. So if you are hard on yourself, unable to love yourself, others will find it hard to give to you and to love you fully.

What you attract starts from within yourself. If you focus on the negative, negativity and difficult situations are what you will get and see. In a nutshell, you see the world not as it is, but from your state of mind. This is why different people can have a different experience and perception of the same event and why we make terrible witnesses.

When you change how you perceive and react to the world, you change how the world reacts to you too.

How to Challenge a Belief

This is another great exercise that is beneficial to do with a friend, as they can be there to prompt you as they recognise their own beliefs

1)Write the belief down. For example, "I need to do everything myself to have it done properly."

2)Write down every piece of proof you have that this belief is true. For example:

- *The dishwasher is not emptied properly.*

- *The secretary never uses the correct grammar.*

- *The cleaner never cleans behind the sofa.*

Keep looking and digging and think outside the box until you run out of proof.

3)Now examine each statement and write down every reason why it is not true.

Think of this exercise like a car. The car is the belief and the engine parts are the proofs. As you disprove the proofs you remove parts of the engine, or shoot holes into it.

Without an engine a car is unable to move and the belief no longer has any power.

Top Tips for Mental Wellbeing

- Be aware of and feel your body, mind, emotions and energy.

- Be mindful and in the 'now.'

- Take responsibility for your own actions.

- Don't 'worry about things outside of your control.

- Reduce the amount of time you spend watching or reading the news.

- Focus on positive events.

- Take a moment to pause regularly throughout your day.

- Set realistic expectations.

- Take action on what you want to do.

- Work on your shadows and defence blocks.

- Practice gratitude, compassion and loving kindness to yourself and not just to others.

- Look for joy in all situations.

- Believe in yourself.

- Get support.

You can only heal limiting beliefs and trauma to a degree by working on your own.

To get a true breakthrough your limiting beliefs need to be felt and witnessed by others, as they come from others and all trauma involves another. The best place to do this is in a safe group.

I run groups on Heart Intelligence face-to-face and online, for more information please contact me at:

www.pamlob.com/contact

CHAPTER 5

The Missing Ingredient That Keeps You Stuck

"A woman in her feminine essence knows that before she walks into a room, all she has to do is choose to feel her compassionate nature, her charm, her wit, her patience, or whatever the moment calls for, and it is with her."

Rachel Jayne Groover

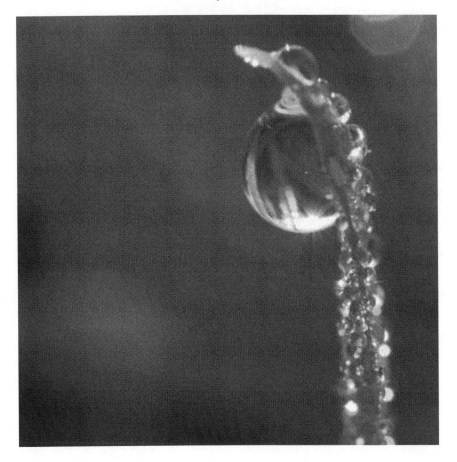

The Missing Ingredient That Keeps You Stuck

WATCH The Missing Ingredient That Keeps You Stuck
http://www.pamlob.com/missing-ingredient

Centuries ago, a few select men in positions of power, within religion and government, were threatened and frightened by the power of women.

They began to do anything possible to keep women's strengths contained. They did this by restricting what a woman was allowed to do, where she was allowed to go, how she could be seen and generally belittling her.

This is still going on today, but it is more apparent in some societies than others.

Here in the west, women have been fighting back over the last hundred years or so. Women started to demand equality, beginning with the Suffragette movement and the right to vote, and by proving women were capable and able to do all kinds of work during the wars.

This was followed by the feminist movement of the 1960's and 70's, fuelled by the sexual freedom the introduction of the contraceptive pill allowed. There is still a way to go and I believe one of the stumbling blocks is women have tried to be equal by copying the behavior of men, instead of using their own amazing feminine essence, strength and acumen.

At the Vancouver Peace Summit in 2009 the Dali Lama said, "The world will be saved by the western woman." He also said, "Some people may call me a feminist... but we need more effort to promote basic human values - human compassion, human affection. And in that respect, females have more sensitivity for others' pain and suffering."

More and more women are rediscovering their feminine essence, their truth, authenticity, strength and power. It is from this place that women are truly able to change the world.

A river is a great analogy of the feminine. A river flows and is the giver of life. It can be soft, gentle, curvaceous, and it can be strong, powerful and even capable of moving mountains.

When a woman is disconnected from her feminine essence, it's as if she is living in a pond and is unable to connect with the flow and ever-changing pleasures of a river. She is unable to be her true self and this unconsciously adds stress to her system.

What is Feminine Essence?

We are energetic beings and our energy has both male and female essences, but one of them will be dominant. This typically goes with gender, so most women have a dominant feminine essence, although a small percentage may feel more comfortable with the masculine essence. (This is not correlated with sexual preference).

Your essence is activated when you make certain physical, energetic and emotional shifts. Not understanding or acknowledging your own, or others' natural essence, leads to misunderstandings and breakdowns in communication. How the two essences respond and react to a situation are vastly different.

Most women have been denying themselves access to their natural feminine essence. Denial or disconnection from your own natural essence leads to stress, health issues, lack of joy and inability to attract and sustain a passionate and loving relationship.

A woman who embodies her feminine essence will have a better sense of herself, more confidence and self-esteem and greater ease in creating lasting love, passion and fulfilment.

Connecting to your feminine essence is not about the clothes you wear, wearing pink, makeup and jewellery, as your essence comes from within. These external props can help you feel more feminine, especially when you practice coming into this way of being. I can feel as feminine in my jeans and wellingtons as I do in a dress and heels.

Feminine essence comes from within, from bringing your awareness into your body, in the 'now' moment and away from your chattering mind. Feminine essence is about joy, emotions and connecting with life. It is about forging relationships rather than logic and competition.

A woman's feminine presence comes from being connected to her feminine essence. A woman who is in her feminine essence is magnetic, radiant and will turn heads when she enters a room as people are automatically drawn to her.

It has nothing to do with how you look on the outside, or what body parts are no longer present. You can still be feminine without breasts or a womb.

Some Masculine and Feminine Essence Traits	
Feminine	Masculine
Body	Head
Emotional	Mental
Flow	Structure
Soft	Hard
Round	Angular
Nurturing	Protective
Being	Doing
Multi-tasking	Focused
Unpredictable	Predictable
Changing	Unchanging
Surrender	Separate
Receptive	Control
Wild	Penetrating
Intuitive	Contained
Seeing the big picture	Pushing
Connection with others	Goal orientated

When you are in tune with your feminine essence, you are connected to your power, able to express your feelings freely and can be guided by your heart, body and intuition towards what you want. You are able to follow your own desires rather than what someone else says you should or must do. You feel joy and pleasure in the small things that happen every day, as your day unfolds from just being, rather than being focused on doing.

Work is less effort and more productive as you are able to be in the moment. You are not wasting energy on feeling guilty about the past, or worrying about the future. It's easier to seek assistance and work cooperatively with others. Relationships can blossom as communication and understanding are improved.

Being feminine is not weaker than masculine, it's just different. Trying to compete with your masculine essence against a man is destined to fail.

Feminine essence is not all about being soft, gentle and floaty. Feminine essence can also be strong and authoritative, the mama bear energy that protects and makes sure everything is all right.

This is not about denying your masculine essence - you need both, but you need more of your dominant essence. You need the polarity of both essences to be charismatic, present and fully alive.

Why Have Women Become Disconnected From Their Feminine Essence?

Women who are currently in midlife transition grew up during the feminist movement of the 1960s and 70s, in which women were fighting for equality and freedom from oppression and male supremacy. This resulted in women believing they are meant to be independent and self-sufficient. It became a matter of pride not to turn to men for help.

I plead guilty to this. It wasn't until after my husband died that I realised I was not doing my friends, my family or myself any favours in always trying to be independent. My husband and I had an amazing relationship. Yet it could have been even better if I had been more connected to my feminine essence, if I had been prepared to be vulnerable and surrender at times.

117

Surrender is not about losing your power or being submissive, it's about going with the flow and being totally in the moment. Despite having had a total hysterectomy and disconnection from my pelvis and 'lady part' due to pain and endless medical intervention, finding my feminine essence has been one of the biggest shifts for me on my personal development journey. It has been truly healing on a physical, emotional and spiritual level.

I now feel connected to who I really am. I feel so much more confident and at ease in my body. I feel in touch with my emotions, energy and intuition. People notice me, in a positive way, and I also feel safer and more relaxed around others.

As I write this I am still looking for a loving relationship to take my exploration of my femininity and self to another level, but I know what I want and I'm not prepared to settle for second best. I want a masculine man who can be king to my queen. I know he's out there somewhere and when the time is right our paths will cross.

Many women believe to get on in the workplace and climb the corporate ladder, the only way to get there is to act like men. This has had a negative effect on women, men and the workplace. Being out of their comfort zone has made many women authoritarian, aggressive and unable to compromise, especially with other women. They often appear supremely confident, yet inside they are paddling wildly, trying to stay afloat.

Equality has progressed significantly over the last fifty years, but it still has a long way to go. The education system and businesses are still mostly run in a way that favours male attributes, which focus on the mind, goals, structure and order. There is nothing wrong with these attributes, but what has been forgotten is biologically, mentally and physically, men and women are different. If both sets of attributes were accepted the world would be healthier, happier and more productive.

As John Gray suggests in his series of books 'Men are from Mars, Women are from Venus,' we might as well be from different planets!

When a woman is disconnected or denying her feminine essence, not only does it have a negative impact on herself, as her spark is missing or dimmed, but men around her are also affected. If a woman is not in her feminine essence, it's hard for a man to step into his masculine essence. The masculine essence naturally wants to provide and protect the feminine. If a woman is being independent, she is denying him this want, dimming his spark and making herself less attractive to him. This is probably what is causing the rise in the use of pornography and sexism against women. This is not saying you should be dependent on men at all times, just that you should sometimes give them the opportunity to show their strengths. So let men hold the door open for you, or move those heavy boxes, or choose where to take you for dinner.

Not only in the working environment, but also at home and in the bedroom, women are denying their feminine essence. They don't want to be perceived as weak and needy, but in doing so they are actually disconnecting from their source of power, magnetism and sensuality. Being authentic and vulnerable can be incredibly powerful. When you are not being true to yourself, you rarely deceive others, only yourself, as your body language will frequently give you away. There is a loss of resonance and harmony between your actions and words, which causes others to withdraw and prevents them from trusting you fully.

Some women may be scared of their feminine essence, as they have been abused or have received unwanted attention from men. However by denying your sexuality in a wholesome, safe way, you potentially invite more of this unwanted attention. By stepping into and knowing how to control the power of your feminine essence, you can feel safe and are able to be your true authentic self.

Connect With Your Feminine Essence

The quickest and easiest way to connect to your feminine essence is through movement. A feminine walk comes more from the hips and has more grace and flow. If you observe men and women walking through town they look very similar, as most women are either in a neutral or masculine essence. When in your masculine essence, the focus is on the chest and shoulders and you are only aware of what is in front of you. Whereas when you are connected with your feminine essence, the connection is with your pelvis, hips and legs. Your upper body is relaxed and you are aware of everything that is going on around you.

If you are in your body and full feminine essence, your body is totally grounded and it is possible to walk fast and purposefully, but still move with grace and ease.

A Simple Practice to Help You Connect to Your Feminine Essence

The powerhouse of your feminine essence is your womb space. This is about three inches below your navel and your hips (it doesn't make any difference if you have had a hysterectomy).

Focus your attention here and let your shoulders and upper body be relaxed.

Allow your breath to go down into your belly, soften your heart and send out love.

Move your hips in any way that feels good to you – back and forth, or in circles.

Now walk around the room, or down the street.

What do you notice?

Women on The Art of Feminine Presence™ courses report that when they are connected to their femininity, they are much more aware of things and people around them. Everything is brighter and more colourful.

Why not practice walking in the feminine as you go into work or around the supermarket? Notice what happens. Please drop me a line on Facebook or Twitter and let me know the results.

I'm sure you have heard the term and experienced 'gut instinct.' Your guts do contain cells similar to those found in the brain and they are of course located in your pelvis. When you take your attention and your breath into your pelvis, you are much more in touch with your intuition and you can silence the little niggling voice in your head. You will feel grounded, calm, confident and peaceful. Listen to your intuition, your gut instinct. It very rarely, if ever, leads you astray.

Before I walk into a room at an event, or before and during getting up to talk, or whenever I have anything difficult to do, I pause for a moment. I take my attention and breath down into my pelvis, I move my hips and I instantly feel calmer, more confident and able to face the task ahead. I highly recommend that you practice this throughout your day, as I'm sure it will help you enormously in all areas of your life.

The more you are connected to your body, emotions and intuition, the more you are able to know what it is you want and what is right for you.

The Costs of Being Disconnected From Your Feminine

In our fast-moving world it's increasingly difficult for women to stay connected to their femininity. But to remain fit and healthy with good relationships, connection is vital.

When a woman is disconnected, life feels like you constantly have to push large rocks up hill, both at work and at home. In contrast, men tend to thrive on pushing these rocks. It has been reported that in the workplace women's stress levels are twice that of men and four times the level in the home.

The cost of being in masculine mode is that you are preventing the production of oxytocin, the feel-good hormone that is helpful in reducing your stress. By being independent and striving to be successful, you produce more testosterone. This can feel good and strong in the short term, but it quickly results in depleted levels of oxytocin and the kick wears off, leaving you feeling even more depleted.

You need testosterone, as it is an important hormone in producing sexual desire. It is also vital for bone strength and muscle density, but like all your hormones it needs to be in balance, or health issues occur.

The way to boost oxytocin is to do something pleasurable.

Pleasure

Life should be pleasurable and joyful. Life can be difficult and chaotic at times, but joy and pleasure can still be found at any time.

One of the quickest ways to reset your body and hormones to normal is through 'heart centred positive emotion.' For women this can be achieved by embracing pleasure. For men it's about being still.

Pleasure is essential for women to maintain their health. It is not something to feel guilty about. Without pleasure the effects of stress increase, you feel sad or depressed and easily agitated. You are more likely to find false pleasure and comfort from alcohol, drugs or junk food.

For many women, when they think of the word 'pleasure' they think of sexual pleasure, but pleasure is so much more. Pleasure is doing something, anything that you enjoy.

It is not possible to have pleasure and stress in the same moment. We have to choose.

Which are you choosing in each moment?

When you are constantly striving, competing, adding to the never ending 'To Do' list, you are working from your masculine essence, which is constantly stressing your body and unbalancing your hormones.

Men de-stress and recharge through stillness, but stillness rarely works for women. Seeing the men in your life veg-ing in front of the TV, or coming home and collapsing into a chair, whilst you are rushing around doing supper and helping the kids with their homework is probably deeply annoying to you. For a peaceful household and to have his cooperation later, allow him this downtime to de-stress and then ask him for assistance and he's much more likely to jump up and help.

For women, pleasure and movement are required to reset and de-stress.

Saida Désiets, author of 'The Succulence Revolution' suggests that most women are barely tapping into the amount of pleasure that they could experience.

Pleasure not only releases oxytocin but also nitrous oxide, a gas within your blood stream which improves blood flow, enabling your body to receive more nutrients and remove waste products. It also causes the production of neurotransmitters, which carry messages around your nervous system. These neurotransmitters improve your mood and help you feel euphoric. In addition, they help to reduce the levels of cortisol that are raised by stress. Pleasure also increases production of the hormone DHEA, which helps balance your oestrogen, progesterone and testosterone levels.

Simply planning and talking about something pleasurable with other women will raise your oxytocin levels, but be careful you use positive language.

For example, saying:

> "I have to go shopping," changes your hormones in the testosterone direction.

> "I'm going shopping," will have a neutral effect.

Whereas saying:

> "Great, I'm going shopping with my girlfriends," will raise your oxytocin.

Pleasure can be:

- Dancing

- Yoga, Pilates, Tai Chi or Qigong

- Movement meditations

- Being out in nature

- A good hug

- Shopping

- Cooking or eating good food

- Wearing/buying beautiful shoes and clothes

- Enjoying everyday things.

The second most important form of pleasure is spending time with female friends. It's sisterhood! These are friends who help you feel alive and energised by spending time in their company. Avoid people who are emotional vampires and leave you needing a nap after spending time with them.

The No.1 type of pleasure that is like hitting a reset button is orgasm. An orgasm that resonates through your body, where climax may or may not happen, but you're totally in the moment with no preconceived goal. This can be alone or with a partner.

Sexuality

Sex is a great way to stay healthy and vibrant.

Having regular sex improves health and wellbeing. It is great for reducing stress and improves circulation and lymphatic drainage, thus stimulating the body's natural detoxification processes. It also improves digestion, which helps protect you against heart disease, cancer and osteoporosis.

Sex causes spikes in the levels of nitrous oxide and the hormone DHEA within your body. This leads to improved brain function, tissue repair and a boosted immune system, which keeps you looking and feeling younger, fitter and healthier.

To feel sexy, sensuous and attractive starts with you. It's how you feel about yourself on the inside.

A woman who is secure in her own sensuality and body is much more attractive to others than the most beautiful model who is not comfortable in her own skin. Likewise, you don't need skimpy clothes, makeup or fancy hair. If you feel attractive and sensuous, people will be drawn to you even if you are wearing a sack.

It's time to stop hiding and to celebrate! Be comfortable with what you've got!

Menopause is not the death bell for sexual experiences. Quite the contrary, as a woman's sex drive can actually increase after menopause.

Sex is available, if you want it, till the day you die. Many seventy and eighty year olds report that sex is now better than ever. Sex after menopause can take on a whole new meaning as it is now for pleasure, without the urgent desire to get pregnant, or the fear of becoming pregnant. It's easier to be relaxed, because as your children get older they are less likely to barge in on you, or want you to be up and about at a ridiculously early hour.

During midlife transition, the brain in both men and women rewires. Often men become more nurturing and more prepared to take their time and offer their partner what they want. Women become more focused on their own needs and more able to ask for what they want. Improved communication and relaxation between a couple can result in more intimacy and a greater enjoyment of sexual relations.

Sex is not just about intercourse with a partner and being there to satisfy them. You don't need to have a partner to connect with your sensuality and enjoy sexual experiences. Culture has led many women to believe their role is to please others, but to be able to totally give to another, first you need to please yourself.

To fill yourself up first!

When we fly in an aeroplane, we are told if there is a sudden decrease in cabin pressure, we should put our oxygen mask on first, so we are able to help others. This is true in all areas of your life. You need to think of YOU first and make your joy and happiness a priority.

When you are responsible for and able to make your own pleasure, you will no longer feel frustrated or disappointed when you don't get what you want from others. You'll stop feeling like a victim and will be in control of your own destiny.

You alone are responsible for turning yourself on.

Enjoy exploring your own body, discover what feels good to you with your clothes on and off. Go out and buy yourself some sexy underwear and wear it every day, not just on special occasions that actually never seem to arise! Invest in a wand or a vibrator and most importantly have fun.

Once you are comfortable with yourself, a partner can assist you and take you to a higher level of pleasure and surrender. Tell your partner what you want, their greatest desire is to please you. Partners aren't mind readers and what they believe may please you is likely to be different from what actually does. Sex can then become a balance of giving and receiving, resulting in limitless joy and pleasure.

Good sex involves the whole of you, not just your sexual organs, but also your mind, body and spirit. Your mind plays a big part in sexual experiences. If you believe sex is only for the young, you are likely to have a low libido and find sex a bit of a chore. Whereas if you think of yourself as a sexual being, deserving and capable of enjoying sex for the rest of your life, this is what will be available.

Having a hysterectomy, mastectomy or even being paralysed from the waist down is not a deterrent from having a pleasurable, stimulating sex life. Even just thinking about sex can lead to an orgasm. Intercourse for a woman is the icing on the cake. Foreplay, kissing, cuddling, stroking all areas of your own and your partner's body, expands and maximises what pleasure means to you. It's not about the goal, or trying to achieve anything. Be in the moment and most importantly enjoy the experience.

Orgasm

Women have an organ purely for pleasure - the clitoris. The clitoris is a small, budlike organ situated just above your vaginal opening and urethra (where you urinate from). The clitoris is made up of 8,000 nerve endings.

When stimulated by touch, the bud swells and you feel sexually excited and ultimately orgasm. It is the main, but not only source of orgasm. There is also the G spot, situated within the vagina. Touch anywhere on your body or even thought can elicit an orgasm if you are in the right frame of mind.

Many women have difficulty in having an orgasm. This may be because they are afraid of, or out of touch with their sensuality, or sex is a rushed job. If you are tense, unable to relax or surrender to the moment, or you see sex as a duty, orgasm is not going to happen, whether pleasuring yourself or with another.

If this is you, be gentle with yourself. Relax and start by just looking at your body in the mirror, or stroking your arms, build up slowly to the rest of your body. Then when you feel ready, put on some soft music and lie in the bath, or on the bed, before gently touching and exploring your womanly parts.

It is good to explore on your own to begin with and find out what feels good to you. Try different types of touch, fast, slow, light, firm, big movements and small movements. Once you feel comfortable, then you can involve your partner in the exploration.

Taking your time and relaxing is the major key. This is not something to be hurried. It is time to relax, have fun and explore, without even having orgasm as a goal.

If you continue to have problems with orgasm or any other sexual issue, you might benefit from speaking to a professional who deals with women's health, or taking a course on intimacy and sexuality.

Vaginal Dryness

If vaginal dryness occurs, it is easily remedied by the use of lubricant. There are several on the market and it is also possible to get oestrogen cream prescribed by your doctor. Personally, I like coconut oil as it is totally natural and hypoallergenic, with antibacterial and antiviral properties.

Playing with a jade egg is another great way to increase lubrication naturally and to tone your vagina at the same time. The jade egg is an egg-shaped piece of jade with a hole drilled through it. Dental floss (replaced after every use) is threaded through the egg to help remove it easily.

Jade is strong and non-porous, so it doesn't harbour bacteria. It heats up to body temperature quickly and also has amazing healing properties. Using a jade egg has many benefits including improved pelvic health, increasing libido, stimulating vaginal secretions, healing incontinence and preventing prolapse.

Support in Connecting With Your Feminine Essence

As a woman you are naturally a social being, therefore the best place to explore and experiment with your feminine essence is with a like-minded group of women. A safe place to do this is by joining an Art of Feminine Presence™ workshop (available worldwide).

These workshops offer a range of exercises to support you in connecting with your feminine essence as well as your body, mind, emotions and spirituality. More information is available at:

http://bit.ly/2AqofBF (This is an affiliate link)

CHAPTER 6

Blueprint to Balance Your Life and Relationships

"Life is really simple, but we insist on making it complicated."
Confucius

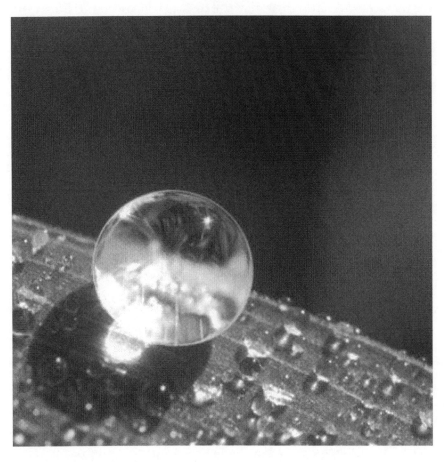

BLUEPRINT TO BALANCE YOUR LIFE AND RELATIONSHIPS

WATCH Blueprint to Balance Your Life and Relationships

http://www.pamlob.com/blueprint-to-balance

Ancient wisdom teaches us the world we see is a reflection of our inner consciousness. Therefore if you want to change your world, you first must change yourself. And this is why I'm here, to support, guide and motivate you to make changes to your life so you are free of menopausal symptoms and have the health, energy and mindset to achieve your hearts desires.

I hear many women say, "I want to be normal."

What is normal? For me, it is something that gets repeated on a regular or daily basis.

Everybody has their own unique view on what is 'normal', so wouldn't it be better and more exciting to say, "I want to be unique!"

Do you really want to start each day thinking, "Oh no, I've got to go to work!" Then screaming at the kids to get out of bed, rushing around preparing breakfast, making packed lunches, finding lost gym shoes, running out the door a few minutes later. Then you're sitting in the car cursing the traffic, dropping the children at school and getting into work already exhausted, frazzled and stressed.

And you haven't even looked at your 'To Do' list yet!

Is This the Type of Life you Really Want?

Have you dreamed about having a job you love? A loving relationship with your partner and children? Having health, energy and balance within your life? Going out and enjoying yourself?

You have the ability to choose the life you want and the capabilities to go for it, if this is what you want.

Your dreams rarely come true from lucky accident. You need to choose what it is you want and take action. The steps only need to be small, so they are not overwhelming.

You only need to take **one small step at a time** to reach your destination! Taking small steps is often more productive and the changes more sustainable, than if you take a giant leap. You don't even need to be sure of what the destination is, you just need to know you want something to change and start to take action.

A great analogy is a satellite navigation system (GPS). It doesn't start working until you start driving. First it needs to be aware of where you are right now (Acceptance). Then it requires a destination. If you are not sure put in any destination that comes to mind as it is taking the action of getting started which is important.

As you get going the destination becomes clearer and clearer. As you start to move the GPS only gives you one step of your journey at a time. Doing this in life prevents overwhelm and confusion. As you journey you are likely to find you have new experiences and new knowledge. You may need to take a diversion, or do a U-turn. These often bring great insight and a recognition that you don't want to go to destination 'A' after all. This is just fine and the way it should be, as life is always full of twists and turns.

Often the reason you have become stressed, overwhelmed or feel lost is because you've continued on blindly to destination 'A' or you've tried to take too many steps at once. Slow down and realise it's ok to divert to destination 'E', or even stop and enjoy the scenery for a while.

The blueprint to taking action and leading a balanced and healthy life, enjoying great relationships and getting rid of menopausal symptoms for good, is to be in the 'River of Life.' When you flow with the river you are connected to who you are, what you are feeling and are mindful of everything and everyone around you.

In the previous chapters I've covered the five most important aspects of a healthy life:

- Reducing Stress

- Eating a healthy diet

- Reducing toxic load

- Being in charge of your mind, not your mind being in control of you.

- Connecting with your feminine essence.

And I've given you some tips and strategies relevant to each topic.

In this next chapter, I share with you some amazing practices, techniques and strategies that have transformed my life and the lives of many of my clients. They can all be easily added to your day and to what you are already doing. Some are as easy as just becoming more aware. All of them will help you feel more relaxed and productive. The reason there are thirteen practices is because this is the sacred energy number of the goddess. It was deemed unlucky in order to control women and undermine their power. I believe it's time for us to reclaim our power and feminine essence and these steps will help you do this.

It can take up to ninety days to change a habit. It involves taking action consciously until it becomes automatic and your subconscious beliefs have changed. It is easy to start out with good intentions, but then life gets in the way and you forget.

Don't beat yourself up if you forget, just start again from where you are. Concentrate on adding just one thing at a time and have it mastered before you move on to the next. Doing it this way you are more likely to succeed and you won't become overwhelmed.

What I find helpful to remember to do new things, is to add them to my diary and put 'post it' notes on the computer, phone, cupboard doors, the fridge and bathroom mirror. Remember to change them regularly so they keep jumping out at you. Setting alarms to remind you to take a pause every 50-60 minutes, or to execute an action, can also be very helpful.

Get yourself an accountability partner or coach to motivate, inspire, support and hold you accountable on this journey. If you are like me you have probably read hundreds of self-help books. Honestly? How much of what you've read you have put into practice?

I know for myself I start off with good intentions and then a couple of weeks later I've forgotten all about it. I have made huge changes in my life over the last few years, on all levels, and it has been working with a coach that has enabled me to make these changes.

I run a program to do just this. If you are interested and looking for a mentor and coach who knows first-hand what it feels like to have horrendous hot flushes, feel overwhelmed, exhausted and unhappy with their weight and looks, get in touch at:

www.pamlob.com/contact

1) Breathe

"There is one way of breathing that is shameful and constricted. Then there's another way; a breath of love that takes you all the way to infinity."
Rumi

Breathing is an essential part of life that is often taken for granted and given little thought. But how you breathe can have a huge effect on your health and wellbeing.

It is commonly believed that we breathe with our lungs alone. In reality breathing involves the whole body, with the lungs playing a passive role in the respiratory process.

Proper breathing involves the muscles of the head, neck, throat and abdomen. Chronic tension in any part of the body, which is common in people who are stressed, affects the natural respiratory movements. Years of sitting at a desk and wearing clothing that is tight around the waist also means that many people don't breathe correctly.

Place a hand on your belly and a hand on your chest and just breathe normally for a few moments.

Don't try to change anything and see what rises and falls the most, your abdomen or your chest? Ideally it should be your abdomen.

Just changing how you breathe even for a few moments can make huge changes to how you feel, especially if you are anxious. This is why yoga and Pilates both focus so much on the breath.

Your mind is unable to focus on two things at once, so when you focus on your breath it allows the chattering voice in your head to be quiet.

What Should Normal Breathing Look Like?

* *Relax.*

* *It's best to breathe in and out of the nose.*

* *Don't force the breath, just let it enter easily and slowly.*

* *You shouldn't hear your breath coming in or out.*

* *Each breath should expand your belly, lower back and ribs.*

* *Relax your shoulders and try not to breathe with your chest.*

* *Put your hands on your stomach and feel them rise and fall.*

* *Focus on stillness and not on forcing an inhale. Your body will breathe when it needs to.*

* *Allow the exhalation to be longer than the inhalation.*

* *Enjoy feeling the good air entering your lungs and feel the stale air leaving your body.*

Keep practising until it becomes natural.

When you are feeling anxious, your normal breath needs a boost with deeper breathing for a few breaths. Too many and you can start to feel dizzy, so three to five is enough. Have the exhalation be longer than the inhalation to reduce dizziness. Then allow your breath to return to a normal rhythm, but maintain focus on your breathing.

Relaxing Breath

- *Relax your shoulders.*
- *Take a deep breath in through your nose for a count of four.*
- *Hold for count of four.*
- *Blow out through pursed lips for a count of six.*
- *And repeat with a count of between four and seven (do what is comfortable for you) up to five times.*

If you are feeling very anxious, the most effective way I've learnt and clients's love is breathing around a rectangle.

Rectangle Breathing

- *Focus on a rectangle, there are always plenty in most indoor environments, pictures, windows, doors, a piece of paper and if there aren't any you can use your hand.*
- *Let your eyes travel around the rectangle with each part of your breath.*
- *Breathe in on the short.*
- *Breathe out on the long, so that your out breath is longer than your in breath.*
- *Pause briefly at each corner.*
- *Do three to five deep breaths to start with and then allow the breath to return to a normal, unforced rhythm.*

Focusing on the rectangle has a hypnotic effect, increasing the effectiveness of the relaxation.

2) Acceptance

"Life is a series of natural and spontaneous changes. Don't resist them; that only creates sorrow. Let reality be reality. Let things flow naturally forward in whatever way they like".
Lao Tzu

Unless you accept what is happening in and with your life, what you resist persists, as life attracts what you put your attention on.

Acceptance is not about liking a situation, it is just recognition that this is how things are right now. When you don't accept something, all you are doing is spending your time and energy on resistance rather than changing the situation. You will never be able to move forward with your life in regard to a situation you are in without acceptance.

Acceptance allows you to see possibilities. It's an agreement with yourself to appreciate, validate, accept and support who you are at this moment. It's an agreement to love yourself, regardless of what else is happening in your life.

Acceptance starts from focusing on what is working in your life and your good qualities. It's about being grateful for the small things that happen or are in your life every day. Progress really begins to happen when you can love and approve of the qualities you think of as 'not good enough.'

What we see as our shadows hide a key to what can be our greatness. That key can come to light when you accept what you see as your darker side, or even your light.

Accepting our good qualities can be as difficult as what we see as our bad. It is our own internal limiting beliefs which cause us to see things as a shadow or to deny them entirely. Others can often see these shadows and don't see them as an issue or problem at all.

Self-acceptance is about releasing other people's opinions of you. You may have been told things, especially in childhood such as, "You can't sing, you are not good enough for the school choir, stop that noise." You carry on believing in adulthood that you can't sing, when in fact you have a beautiful voice. Even if it's not pitch perfect and you might not be the next Adele, if you want to sing, you should sing.

Sometimes we may think we know what someone else is thinking, or saying about us, but most of the time it's not true. How often do you think negative thoughts or judgments about another? My guess is not often, so why are you thinking that others are thinking bad thoughts about you?

Do you want to feel good?

Acceptance and loving yourself is the key.

A client came to see me who was struggling with anxiety and panic attacks. She had come to associate the panic attacks with being hot. She was having frequent hot flushes and every time she had one it brought up a feeling of panic. The panic attacks also began to happen whenever she was hot. This was affecting all areas of her life, including making her reluctant to go on holiday.

We worked on learning to disassociate being hot from the feeling of panic. Her real breakthrough was accepting at times it was just hot, even if the heat came from a hot flush. Even now, several years later, she still tells me that she hears my voice in her head saying, "It's just hot!"

3) Pause: Find Inner Stillness

"Be still. Stillness reveals the secrets of eterniy"
Lao Tzu

To be able to change, first you need to be aware of what you want to change. Often when you are deep within an issue, you cannot see or recognise what is going on. It can be obvious to a third party, but not to you.

Your level of stress and how much it is impacting on your life has just become 'normal'! To be able to recognise what is going on, you need time to take stock of all areas of your life. The best way to do that is to take time to 'pause.'

Life is never still. Change is happening moment by moment as time passes by. Control is just an illusion! Fundamentally, if nothing changed, nothing could happen and reality would be frozen forever.

Today's frenetic lifestyle, which encourages striving for the next bright bauble, allows very little time for pause, for stillness or for just being.

How often in your day do you pause and take time to just be still, or connect with your inner wisdom and intuition?

My guess is your answer is rarely or not at all.

Society and upbringing in western culture trains and encourages us to live our lives from our headspace, our mind.

But our mind is only about 10% of who we are. We also have a body, emotions, energy, intuition, which are rarely used to anywhere near their full potential. They are quite likely just taken for granted and ignored, if you live from your head and not your heart.

Pausing allows you to have the space to listen to your body, emotions, energy and intuition. It allows you to recognise what you want and what action you need to get there. This clarity reduces overwhelm, as you are clear on each step, rather than bouncing from one thing to another to see what will work, or even worse are multitasking.

You don't need all the answers, just what the next step is. As you take each step, your destination becomes clearer.

Pause

Take time to pause and tune in with yourself regularly throughout your day. It only needs to be for a minute or two.

- *Pause between tasks, after 50 minutes focused work, whilst waiting for the kettle to boil, or whilst standing in a queue.*

Close your eyes (if it is safe to do so) and take your attention to your breath. If you are out in nature focus on a tree branch dancing in the wind, or the flow of water in a river or stream.

Next move your attention to your body.

- *How is your body feeling right now?*
- *Do you have any pain or discomfort?*
- *Are you tense in your shoulders or knees?*

Be inquisitive! Whatever is there is ok. Nothing is wrong, it's just how it is right now.

Now move your attention to your emotions.

- *What are you feeling right now?*
  Happy, sad, angry, frustrated?

Sometimes emotions are felt physically.

- *If you are feeling sad, you may feel a heaviness in your heart or solar plexus.*
- *If you are angry, you might feel tension in your jaw or shoulders.*

Whatever you feel is ok. Likewise if you don't feel anything, that is also fine.

As you focus your awareness on your body and emotions, be aware of any judgements or stories that might arise in your mind. Just acknowledge them and return your focus to your breath, or body.

As you give yourself time in this space, it gives your intuition time to give you a pop up that can be heard, felt or seen. You may recieve answers you have been searching for, guidance on your next step in what you are working on, or even the next step in life..

Listen and download Pause
http://www.pamlob.com/pause/

I have found that by adding regular pauses in my day,
I am more relaxed. I am more in tune with and able to hear what my body, emotions and energy are telling me and in turn, I am more productive. I'm sitting writing this in bed with regular pauses to watch the tree dancing outside my window. I have found that when I sit at the computer, words rarely flow.

Start adding moments of pause throughout your day. Just stop what you are doing, especially if you are feeling stuck or frustrated, and take a few moments to tune in with yourself. See what a difference it makes to your life. If you are out in nature, pause and soak up your surroundings. Feel replenished by the elements.

4) Gratitude

"Reflect upon your present blessings – of which every man has many – not on your past misfortunes, of which all men have some.
Charles Dickens

A major part of being fit and well is how you think and feel about things going on in your life. A positive outlook can make you look and feel fit and healthy. It plays a major part in curing or reducing health issues.

One of the most effective strategies to change a negative mindset is gratitude. It is probably the number one favourite exercise for my clients to reduce pessimism, worry and stress.

Gratitude increases positivity, because it helps balance the scales between giving and receiving. Women especially are experts at meeting the needs of others but not their own. If someone pays us a compliment, we often dismiss it with a negative comment.

Most people don't notice the millions of things to be grateful for in each day. Our brain is biased to focus on the negative and not the positive, unless we train it otherwise.

Practice Gratitude

Treat yourself to a small notebook.

Each night before you go to sleep write down five things you are grateful for that day.

No Repeats

If you are struggling, look at all areas of your life and what is going on in your environment e.g. I am grateful...

- *It was sunny today.*

- *For the compliment I received from ... on how my*

hair/dress looked.

* *I was able to get all the shopping I needed.*

* *My home feels warm and safe on these dark nights.*

* *My son shared what he had done at school today.*

*

Going to sleep with a positive mind helps you to wake up with a positive mind.

The energy you put out into the universe is what you will attract. Therefore, putting out a positive energy means you will receive more positive energy in return.

The action of writing down the things you are grateful for ignites a thought process focused on how you can take action to achieve what you want in life.

Within a few days of doing this exercise you will become more aware throughout each day of little things that make you smile and feel good.

5) Love Yourself

"Your task is not to seek for love, but merely to seek and find all the barriers within yourself that you have built against it"
Rumi

"I love myself." Are you able to say these three words and mean it?

Many people really struggle with this and in the past, I did too.

Why is it so difficult?

From a young age, you are led to believe love is all about others. You give love to them and they give love to you in return.

We have been given the wrong information!

Everything starts with you. You are an energetic being and it is the vibration you put out into the world that determines how others feel about you, how you feel about them and what you attract into your life.

In order to put love out into the world, you first need to feel love within. By loving yourself, you shine more brightly and are able to give so much more to others, especially if your actions come from a place of wanting to give rather than feeling you have to, or should give.

In return, when you are not loving yourself it is difficult to receive and accept the love from others and you are more likely to attract negativity. By not loving yourself you are at the centre of a vicious circle.

You have the freedom to choose your thoughts, so choose ones that are beneficial to you!

Your emotions and feelings come from your thoughts, so if you're thinking negative thoughts it's difficult to feel love. Just changing a thought to the words 'I love myself' several times a day can have a profound, positive effect on how you feel about yourself and the world around you.

I Love Myself Practice

Look at yourself in a mirror and say, "I love you (your name)"

Do this each morning as you get up and each evening as you go to bed.

If you find this too difficult, start with, "I accept myself," or try loving a part of you such as, "I love my eyes."

Gradually add in more parts of you, until you are able to say, "I love you."

If you find that as you look in the mirror you hear judgments and criticism, be aware that the mirror is not making these judgments or criticisms. Your inner thoughts love to tell stories and keep you playing small.

You can change your thoughts and make them more positive.

You will not only change your experience with the mirror, but also your experiences in life. To begin with it may feel like you are lying to yourself, but persevere, it will be well worth it.

Loving and accepting who you are gives you value, safety and trust within yourself and with others. It helps you feel more positive, less stressed and healthier. You are more able to give love to others and attract loving relationships, a better job, and the life of your dreams in return.

Unconditional love for self is the most powerful tool for self-confidence and self- esteem.

6) 'Me time'

"Time is a created thing. To say, 'I don't have time,' is like saying, 'I don't want to.'"
Lao Tzu

A large part of loving yourself and boosting your self-worth is having regular 'me time.' This is time purely for you and is **not** time with the family, or your partner, even though this feeds you and brings you joy.

To be a healthy, whole, authentic human being, you need time alone to replenish and recognise what your body, mind, emotions, energy and intuition wants. Being at the constant demand of others does not give you space to really feel.

Many women believe that putting themselves first is wrong. It is egotistical. However, if you never put your own feelings and needs first, you will eventually not be in a fit state to help others. Just as when you fly you are to put on your own oxygen mask first in an emergency, so that you are able to help others, in everyday life you also need to nourish yourself to have the strength to give.

In life, you need a balance of giving and receiving. Taking vital 'me time' is essential, not a luxury. This may be at an exercise class, a regular massage or reflexology treatment, a relaxing bath, or curling up with a good book. It doesn't have to be for long periods of time, as small short bursts during your day can be extremely beneficial. Such as an extra five minutes alone in bed with a cup of tea before starting the day, a short walk at lunchtime, or coming in from work or the school run and sitting down before starting the supper, chores and homework. It's not only giving you a break, but other family members as well.

Put 'me time' into your diary. If you can't make the time you set, don't just delete it from your diary, move it to another time slot.

'Me time' is **non-negotiable** except in dire emergencies.

YOU ARE WORTH IT!

7) Sleep Well

"Now, blessings light on him that first invented sleep! It covers a man all over, thoughts and all, like a cloak; it is meat for the hungry, drink for the thirsty, heat for the cold, and cold for the hot. It is the current coin that purchases all the pleasures of the world cheap, and the balance that sets the king and the shepherd, the fool and the wise man, even."
Miguel de Cervantes, Don Quixote

Sleep is a natural part of everyone's life. Sleep is a required activity, not an option. We spend about one-third of our lives asleep. Even though the precise functions of sleep remain a mystery, sleep is important for normal motor and cognitive function.

Don't listen to those people who boast, "I only need four hours' sleep a night." This is not something to be proud of, as in the long term, their health will suffer. Most people need about eight to ten hours of good quality sleep to function optimally.

If you are having difficulty in falling asleep or wake up in the middle of the night, the trick to going to sleep, is not trying to sleep. What is most likely to keep you awake is the longing to sleep, because you need to be alert in the morning. The more you try, the less likely it is you will fall asleep.

How to Have a Good Night's Rest

Before Bed:

- *Stick to a regular bedtime routine.*

- *Avoid exercising within four hours of going to bed.*

- *Avoid eating late.*

- *Don't check or send emails in the hour before going to bed.*

- *Keep a notebook beside your bed to jot down anything that suddenly comes to mind and is keeping you awake.*

- *Have a warm (not too hot) bath with relaxing oils such as lavender.*

- *Don't drink too much alcohol. You may fall asleep easily, but are likely to wake in the middle of the night. Sleep is less restful if you have been drinking. The hangover is not just the alcohol!*

If you can't sleep:

- *Don't try to sleep. Be OK with being awake, because if you are trying to sleep, you are resisting being awake and what you resist, persists!*

- *Take your awareness to your body and do some progressive muscle relaxation where you tighten and release your muscles from your feet upwards.*

- *Focus on your breathing. Breathe in slowly right down into your abdomen, and out slowly. Count this as 'one', repeat five times and then start again at one.*

- *If your mind is full of thoughts write them down. This can be done in the dark as it's the act of writing that matters, not whether it makes sense or is neat and tidy.*

- *Listen to a meditation, relaxing music, a radio talk show or audio book.*

- *Put drops of lavender oil on your pillow, or on a tissue so you can breathe in the aroma.*

- *If you are wide awake, get up and make yourself a*

warm drink. Don't do anything stimulating other than reading a few pages of a book or listening to soothing music.

Do not look at anything on your phone or any electronic devises.

Then settle yourself back down to sleep.

8) Learn to say no

*"A '**No**' uttered from the deepest conviction is better than a 'Yes' merely uttered to please, or worse, to avoid trouble."*
Mahatma Gandhi

Saying 'No' can be immensely difficult for some people. It was something I struggled with for many years. Constantly saying 'Yes' does not honour you and can leave you worn out, depleted and unable to serve anyone successfully.

Saying no is not being rude, nor is it a rejection of the person who asked, if the refusal is polite. We often don't say no in the fear of losing friendships, or being thought less of by our boss or work colleagues. Saying no is empowering and can be seen as a sign of strength, not weakness, as long as it's not done from a place of spite. Does it bother you when someone says no to you?

Saying no is a major part of loving yourself. A 'yes' when you really want to say 'no' is saying 'no' to yourself

To be more comfortable in saying "No":

- *Take a moment before responding and feel into yourself to check whether what is being asked is right for you right now, or whether you are comfortable in doing it, or not.*
  Listen to your intuition.

- *Thank the person for asking you.*

- *A simple "No" or "I can't right now" is sufficient. But if it makes you more comfortable, you can follow up with "Good luck in finding someone," or "Please think of me if you need someone in the future."*

- *Practice.*

We have the choice to say "Yes" or the choice to say "No". Always saying "Yes" diminishes it's meaning as it's not done from choice. Regain your power and choice today by learning to say "No."

9) Receiving

"A generous man forgets what he gives and remembers what he receives."
Old Proverb

Imagine an old pair of scales, you know, the ones where you add weights to a tray on either side of a balance arm. Now add a weight for each time you've done something for someone else onto one side. On the other side, add a weight for every time you've received a gift, a compliment, or some help.

My guess is the scales are out of balance, with the giving side unable to take any more weight!

Being caring, giving and independent has its virtues, but it can also be a defence against receiving. It's not the way to lead a healthy balanced life. You also need to be the recipient.

As already discussed, to be able to give you need to fill yourself up first. Another way of filling yourself up is receiving with grace.

What do I mean by 'receiving with grace'?

When you receive a compliment on how you look or what you are wearing, how often do you reply with, "Oh it's old," or, "It only came from a bargain store," or, "Actually, I need to get a haircut."

A compliment is a gift, but if you answer back in this way, it is not 'receiving with grace' but literally throwing the gift back at the giver. Receiving with grace is pausing and then saying, "Thank you!" and nothing more.

If you struggle with asking for help, or receiving offers of help, consider for a moment your response to someone asking you for help. If it's possible to help someone, the answer is likely to be yes. If you see a friend struggling, do you offer help? How do you feel if it's rejected?

Helping is a gift to the recipient, but giving is also a gift to the giver. By not accepting help, you are denying the joy of giving to another.

Giving is only a gift to you, the donator, if it feels good, doesn't deplete you and is something you want to do. If it's not, say "No". This is much more of a gift and is more authentic than saying "yes" from a place of resistance.

10) Be Mindful and Heart Centred

"Each morning we are born again. What we do today is what matters most."
Buddha

Are you aware of the beauty of sunlight glistening through a raindrop, the smile of appreciation from a work colleague, or the energy that flows constantly through your body?

The stresses of modern life have meant that most people are disconnected from themselves and from the world around them. Many move through the day feeling guilty about the past, worrying about tomorrow's meeting or what to cook for dinner. I call this living from your headspace and as I've already mentioned, but cannot emphasis enough, you are so much more.

Mindfulness is …

- Being in the present moment.

- Awareness of what is going on around you.

- Being aware of how your body feels, what your emotions are and what your intuition is telling you in any given moment.

By being mindful of what is happening around you and within you, it is possible to recognise what it is you need or want right now. This doesn't have to be some big goal, it can be as simple as giving a hug, wanting a cup of tea or standing and enjoying your surroundings.

Mindfulness has been found to reduce depression and anxiety and has a positive effect on many health issues. Focusing on what is going on around you or what you are doing can be a helpful way to deal with pain. If you feel your mind wandering off into yet another story or judgment, just bring your awareness back to the present moment and focus on what is happening around you and within you.

Being heart centred is an extension of mindfulness. Our heart is the centre of our emotional and spiritual being and is the first thing that forms at birth. When you live from your heart, you are being authentic to who you truly are. You're not putting on an act to fit in with how others think you should behave. Not everyone is going to like you, whichever road you take, but being authentic is relaxing for you and very attractive to another. When you are aware, you can always tell when someone is being inauthentic.

Listen to what your body, emotions, energy and intuition are telling you. Learn to feel more.

Can you feel your energy?

Rub your hands together and then hold them about an inch apart.

Can you feel the buzz between them? This is your energy. It is energy that you are reading when you feel that someone is inauthentic.

When you feel your mind wandering in the present or back into the past, bring your awareness back to the now.

Feel your body, emotions and energy.

Become fully aware of what is happening around you.

Begin to see the beauty that is all around you and feel less exhausted, less stressed and less confused.

11) Meditation and Relaxation

"What is this true meditation? It is to make everything: coughing, swallowing, waving the arms, motion, stillness, words, action, the evil and the good, prosperity and shame, gain and loss, right and wrong, into one single koan."

Hakuin

The purpose of meditation is to relax, to reduce stress and cortisol levels. It helps you to get more in touch with your body, improve your mood and quieten the chatter in your head. All of which can help to reduce hot flushes and improve sleep and memory function. Meditation also helps you feel happier and it allows space for your intuition to be heard and creativity to develop.

Meditation is not about trying to silence your mind. It's about focusing your attention, which allows you to quieten your mind. The attention may be on your breath, on your body, on a candle, the sound of someone's voice, or the feeling of the ground beneath your feet.

Meditation does not have to be sitting cross legged on the floor, like an Indian guru. It can be done in any position, even walking. In fact, walking, focusing on how my body is feeling and the feel and sound of each footfall, is one of my favourite ways to meditate. It is a good place for a beginner to start.

A very powerful mediation and another of my favourites, helps you connect with your body and your feminine essence.

Put on a slow piece of music without words.

Then in a standing position, focus on one part of your body, such as your arm.

Gradually and slowly begin to move your arm in any way that feels good to you.

Explore how slow you can go and what range of movement you can do.

155

Sometimes, just pause in a position and wait until you feel your body wants to move again. When you feel ready, move on to another part of your body and repeat.

You can also take your attention down to your pelvis, womb space and hips. Try different movements and see what you enjoy and find relaxing.

If thoughts come into your head acknowledge them and return your focus to the part of your body you are moving. Enjoy!

There are hundreds of guided meditations and relaxations available. There are also meditations that have been recorded in specific frequencies with binaural beats, that can help you go into a deeper brain wave state. Always listen before purchasing, as some people's voices, accents and the speed of their vocal delivery might not be for you. It may irritate, rather than relax you.

Find a time in the day that works well for you. I find first thing in the morning works best for me. I listen to a recorded mediation before I get up, as at night I'm likely just to fall asleep.

I then do a walking meditation as I walk the dog and a feminine essence meditation before going to a meeting, or recording a video. In fact, I do this meditation anytime I want to be in my feminine power.

12) Exercise

"An early-morning walk is a blessing for the whole day."
Henry David Thoreau

Exercise is vital for your health and wellbeing. It can help you lose weight, keeps your joints supple, your muscles strong, boosts your immune system, improves your mood, reduces stress, helps prevent osteoporosis and can reduce the symptoms of the menopause and ageing.

Many people think of exercise as going to the gym and pounding away on a treadmill, pumping weights, or doing an exhausting hour of aerobics. If you enjoy these and feel they are benefiting your body - great, however they are not for everyone. For optimal results it's advisable to do the right type of exercise and at the right time of day for your body type.

Exercise should be part of your normal day. The NHS in the UK is challenging everyone to walk 10,000 steps a day. This can be part of your normal day, as well as going out for a walk.

- If you drive, park further away from work, or the supermarket entrance.

- If you catch the bus or train, get off a stop earlier.

- Take the stairs as often as you can. Stairs not only add to your steps, but raise your heartbeat as well.

- After every 50 minutes of focused work, get up and walk around. Not only is it adding to your step count, but you will be more productive.

- Doing housework can also be energetic, if you want it to be.

Formal exercise should be enjoyable, as if it's not, you are unlikely to keep doing it. There is so much choice, so it's about finding something that you enjoy and is right for your body type.

Exercising can also be vital 'me time' so add it to your diary. Take ten to fifteen minutes at lunchtime, more if possible, and go for a walk. You will feel energised and will be more productive than if you had continued to sit at your desk.

Everyone needs cardiovascular exercise that raises the heart rate at least three times a week. This can be going for a run, doing an aerobic or dance class, but a brisk walk, or walking up hill, or putting on your favourite piece of music and dancing can be as effective. Research has shown that intensive cardiovascular workouts can damage the heart, especially if there are no rest days.

Flexibility is important as you age, to keep your joints supple and prevent injury. Simple stretching exercises can be performed at home, but initially I would recommend going to a pilates, or yoga class with a qualified instructor to learn the correct techniques and prevent injury.

Avoid huge classes at a gym, where the instructor only stands at the front and pushes you beyond your safe limits. In a small class you will learn how to do the movements safely and what is right for your body. Don't be afraid to walk away from a class that does not feel right for you.

Strength training is needed to boost muscle mass. It helps with how you look overall, as well as helping to prevent osteoporosis. Weight training is not the only way. Walking can not only improve your lower body, but your upper body too if you're carrying hand weights, or even shopping bags.

Pilates, Yoga and Tai Chi are an excellent way to build strength and flexibility if you don't want a high impact class. They are slow, as they are very controlled and focused on your breathing, but they offer a good cardiovascular workout too.

One of my favourite forms of exercise that I've recently discovered is 'Rebounding' on a small trampoline. It is great in helping improve lymphatic drainage, so helps to detoxify your body. It also boosts immune function, improves cardiovascular fitness and even helps with getting rid of that stubborn cellulite, without placing any stress on the joints. Just a few minutes each day is all you need. It can be done whilst watching the TV or out in the garden. Research by NASA has found that it can be twice as effective as running on a treadmill.

If you want to know the right exercises for your body type contact me:
http://www.pamlob.com/contact

13) Connecting with Nature

"I remember a hundred lovely lakes, and recall the fragrant breath of pine and fir and cedar and poplar trees. The trail has strung upon it, as upon a thread of silk, opalescent dawns and saffron sunsets. It has given me blessed release from care and worry and the troubled thinking of our modern day."

Hamlin Garland

Connecting with nature on a daily basis has been shown to reduce depression, boosting energy and wellbeing.

I find going for a walk each day with the dog always boosts how I feel. Even on a grey, wet day, I come back feeling refreshed and energised.

You don't need a dog, or to have countryside on your doorstep to connect with nature. Even in the city, you are never far from a green space.

Nature is there to rebalance your senses. It asks for nothing in return.

It is easy in your busy life to take what nature there is around you for granted and not really take any notice of it.

I invite you to take some time every day to pause, be mindful and enjoy whatever nature there is around you, even if it's just the sky.

On your way to work and on your way home spend a few minutes in a park, or green space, or looking up at the sky. Preferably somewhere away from roads and motor vehicles. At lunchtime get away from your desk and go outside if only for a few minutes. You will be much more productive than if you stay sitting at your desk.

Be mindful and focus on the beauty around you, rather than the voice in your head that is worrying, or feeling guilty. Instead, take your awareness to each of your senses in turn.

Listen to the sound of birds or the wind rustling the leaves of a tree. Enjoy feeling the breeze and the sun on your skin, smell the fragrance of any flowers or newly mown grass.

160

See the different colours and tones of the grass, the sky and whatever else is around you.

Bring nature inside. Sit by a window if possible, have plants on your desk and around your home, treat yourself to some fresh flowers, or ask your partner to treat you to some.

Another option is to place pictures on your desk of somewhere beautiful which makes you feel relaxed.

Start connecting with the nature around you today. We are all part of the natural world and connecting with it can have a huge beneficial effect on your life, your health and the health of this beautiful planet we call home.

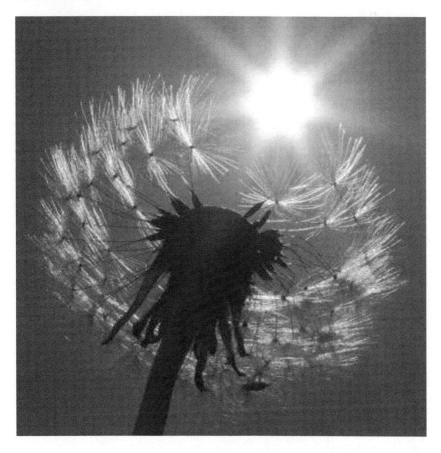

These are just a few practices to get you started in living in the 'River of Life' and improving your health, wellbeing and relationships.

If you want to learn more and in greater depth, or need support and motivation please contact me at:

http://www.pamlob.com/contact

References

Boardman, H.M.P et al; (2015) Hormone Therapy For Preventing Cardiovascular Disease In Post-Menopausal Women. Cochrane Library.

Lee. J.R, Hopkins. V., (2004) What Your Doctor May Not Tell You About Menopause. Grand Central Publishing, New York.

Perlmutter, David; (2015) BrainMaker: The Power of Gut Microbes to Heal and Protect Your Brain. Little, Brown and Company, New York.

Pesticide Action Network. (2015) http://www.pan-uk.org/food/best-worst-food-for-pesticide-residues

Scott-Mumby, Keith; (2005) Diet Wise, Toxic Foods are Common and Cause a Lot of Harm. Everyone is Different. Find Out Yours. Mother Whale Inc, Nevada.

INTERACTIVE RESOURCES OVERVIEW

Contact me:
http://www.pamlob.com/contact

Invitation from the author:
http://beyondhotcrazy.gr8.com/

My Story
http://www.pamlob.com/my-story

The Key to an Extraordinary Life
http://www.pamlob.com/key-
extraordinary-life

River of Life Meditation
http://www.pamlob.com/river-of-life/

How to Understand your Raging Hormones
http://www.pamlob.com/understand
raging hormones

Kate's Menopausal Story
http://www.pamlob.com/kates-story/

Jocelyn's Menopause Story
http://www.pamlob.com/jocelyns-story

Elizabeth's Menopause Story
http://www.pamlob.com/elizabeths-story

Are You Addicted to Stress
http://www.pamlob.com/are-you-addicted-
to-stress/

Playbook-Are You Addicted to Stress?
http://www.pamlob.com/are-you-addicted-
to-stress
playbook1

You are what you Eat!
http://www.pamlob.com/you-are-what-
you-eat/

A Food Diary
http://www.pamlob.com/food-diary/

Asea Website
http://pamlob.teamasea.com/

Personalised health webpage
http://www.pamlob.com/personalised-
health.

Why Your Beliefs are Sabotaging You
http://www.pamlob.com/why-your-beliefs/

The Missing Ingredient That Keeps You Stuck
http://www.pamlob.com/missing-ingredient

The Art of Feminine Presence Website
http://bit.ly/2AqofBF (This is an affiliate link)

Blueprint to Balance Your Life and Relationships
http://www.pamlob.com/blueprint-to-balance

Pause meditation
http://www.pamlob.com/pause/

Additional resources
http://www.pamlob.com/resources

Acknowledgements

Bringing this book to fruition is a childhood dream come true. It would not have been possible without help from some very special people.

Thank you from the bottom of my heart to Rachel Jayne Groover (founder of Art of Feminine Presence™) and Christian Pankhurst (founder of Heart IQ™) for transforming my life to one of joy and connection to my body, soul and feminine essence. These remarkable and unexpected changes have given me the courage and determination to write and complete this book.

Thank you also to both communities for providing me with worldwide friendships that have provided ongoing support during the highs and lows of producing this book and in life in general. Names too numerous to mention, but they know who they are.

I am also extremely grateful to Rachel Jayne for honoring me by writing the foreword as well as being a friend and mentor as I take baby steps into the world of business.

A special thank you also for the Regal Squirrel Chicks, my business mentorship group that have become family: Amara Hamilton, Miyuki Miura, Pat McLeod and Lisa Markman, who have tirelessly listened to my ideas, have critiqued my drafts and offered endless encouragement.

Thank you to Sue Hennell for proof reading my first draft and correcting my dyslexic English and to Fay Marcroft of Fay Marcroft PR for editing the first edition and Karen Collyer, www.karencollyer.com for editing the second edition.

Lastly a big thank you to Miyuki Miura of Inspirational Nature Pictures, http://www.inspirationalnaturepictures.com for allowing me to use her beautiful dewdrop pictures throughout this book.

From my heart to yours

Pam Lob

Biography

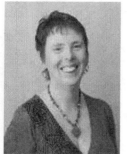 Pam Lob's world turned upside down when her husband died, following her own tiresome and lengthy battle with health issues. It would have been easy for her to hide away from the world and grieve, living a staid and boring existence while carrying on a losing battle with her hormones.

She instead chose to grasp life with both hands, and over the last few years has transformed into a joyfully sassy, healthy, and adventurous goddess who no longer plays small.

As an author, speaker, and 'health genie,' Pam supports and inspires women struggling with health issues, menopause, weight problems, stress, and anxiety— women who would much rather feel healthy, joyful, energised, and fulfilled.

As a qualified nurse, holistic hypnotherapist, counsellor, and coach with a degree in psychology — along with years of personal development and life experience — Pam knows what works. She is not your usual health practitioner who takes a one-size-fits-all approach. She has a unique combination of strategies and secrets to share.

Pam is an international speaker who has appeared on stage and radio in the UK, USA, and Australia. She was featured in the 2014 Bounce Back Queens World Summit.

If you are looking for a speaker on any health matters, please contact Pam at http://www.pamlob.com/contact

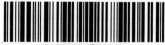

Made in the USA
San Bernardino, CA
12 July 2018